Praise for *Finding Lina*

"In this honest memoir, Hjalmarsson (a psychoanalyst with a master's degree in child development) conveys the frustrations and the triumphs of raising an autistic daughter. She also explains how a special-needs kid affects the rest of the family. . .The family tries everything, including acupuncture, herbal remedies, and dietary changes, while Hjalmarsson remains remarkably positive. 'She taught me to take life as it is,' she writes. 'She showed me how to be happy and laughing in the midst of sorrow and loss.' A passionate book for families with special-needs children."—Karen Springen, *Booklist*

"The author's positive, optimistic attitude and her thorough descriptions of therapies will be helpful to the parents and caretakers of autistic children."—*Kirkus Reviews*

"An inspirational and brave story of Helena's journey to help her daughter. A positive reminder that we learn so much from our children and that each one shines in their own special way. —Jenny McCarthy, bestselling author, activist, and actress

"Not only a mother's painfully honest account of coming to terms with her daughter's autism, but an offering of insight and new possibility to parents facing similar situations, This is a story that resonates beyond the specific illness, with a universality both heart-rending and inspiring."—Dick Russell, *New York Times* bestselling author

"*Finding Lina*'s charm is its laser focus on what it means to accept and be nourished by life's brutal realities--how deep connections require you to truly listen, rather than just to hear, and to keep looking, even when you can't see. This isn't a book about autism, this is a love story."—Jeni Decker, author of *I Wish I Were Engulfed in Flames*

"A gritty, real, intense immersion into autism. You find yourself not as a distant reader but living in the minds and hearts of the parents and the unspeakable discomfort of trying to anticipate and hold the confusion of this problem. The book is a living testimony to overcoming in order to make the family whole and turning suffering into joy."—Leslie Stein, author of *Becoming Whole*

"Plato said of the journey of life that 'the first and best victory is to conquer self.' Those of us with a child on the spectrum are instructed in this maxim. In *Finding Lina*, Hjalmarsson takes us on a journey of transformation with heart and honesty, applicable to not only the challenges of autism but to the trials life hands us all." —Ken Siri, author of *1,001 Tips for the Parents of Autistic Boys* and co-author of *Cutting Edge Therapies for Autism*

"I love how Hjalmarsson completely dispels the theory of the 'refrigerator mother.' She also depicts with grace how she gathers and coordinates the army of people needed to support one special needs child. Hjalmarsson is an inspiration!"—Professor Gayle DeLong, Baruch College, City of University of New York

"A brave and honest book about the journey of one family to overcome the challenge of autism and to build a life of meaning for the child they love."—Louis Conte, board member, Elizabeth Birt Center for Autism Law and Advocacy

"An honest and insightful account of a mother's terrifying and courageous odyssey searching for answers, and ultimately discovering solutions all in the name of her precious daughter, Lina. For anyone who has been through a soul-shaking tragedy, *Finding Lina* is a testament to the power of the human spirit. Helena's unwavering determination demonstrates how one's love for a child can ignite a deep and powerful strength, capable of battling any beast—even autism."—Mary Coyle, Homeopath and Director of the Real child Center

"*Finding Lina* is a poignant narrative of a mother's struggle to lovingly care for a daughter with severe health challenges. The book is at once heartwarming and heartrending, faithfully depicting the extraordinary world of autism parenting."—Mary Holland, co-founder, the Elizabeth Birt Center for Autism Law and Advocacy (EBCALA); co-editor, *Vaccine Epidemic*

"This book is intense and I can only marvel at how much can be asked of a parent. I'm sure much of Helena's strength comes from her deep spiritual beliefs and from being a dedicated mother who knows she can never stop. Just as *Diary of a Young Girl* about Anne Frank put a human face on the Holocaust, books like *Finding Lina* reveal the truth about what autism can do to a child. I just wonder how many more books like this will have to be written before we finally wake up. —Anne Dachel, Media Editor, *Age of Autism* and author of *The Big Autism Cover-Up*

"A poignant look at life raising a daughter on the spectrum and how the entire family unit is affected by the epidemic. And how a family raises above it."—Kim Stagliano, author of *All I Can Handle* and *101 Tips for the Parents of Girls with Autism*

"*Finding Lina* is a story of undaunted courage, hope and love. Parents of children with special needs will be gripped by the honest portrayal of what families endure under unimaginable circumstances. All readers will be drawn into the herculean effort to find answers that lead to a healthier, more fulfilling life."—Mary Romaniec, autism advocate, and author of *Victory Over Autism*

Finding Lina

Finding Lina

A MOTHER'S JOURNEY FROM AUTISM TO HOPE

Helena Hjalmarsson, M.A., L.C.S.W., L.P.

Foreword by Rupert Isaacson, author of
The Horse Boy: A Memoir of Healing

Preface by Amanda Friedman, Director,
Emerge & See Education Center

Skyhorse Publishing

Copyright © 2013, 2016 by Helena Hjalmarsson

All Rights Reserved. No part of this book may be reproduced in any manner without the express written consent of the publisher, except in the case of brief excerpts in critical reviews or articles. All inquiries should be addressed to Skyhorse Publishing, 307 West 36th Street, 11th Floor, New York, NY 10018.

Skyhorse Publishing books may be purchased in bulk at special discounts for sales promotion, corporate gifts, fund-raising, or educational purposes. Special editions can also be created to specifications. For details, contact the Special Sales Department, Skyhorse Publishing, 307 West 36th Street, 11th Floor, New York, NY 10018 or info@skyhorsepublishing.com.

Skyhorse® and Skyhorse Publishing® are registered trademarks of Skyhorse Publishing, Inc.®, a Delaware corporation.

Visit our website at www.skyhorsepublishing.com.

10 9 8 7 6 5 4 3 2 1

Cover designed by Brian Peterson

Library of Congress Cataloging-in-Publication Data is available on file.

ISBN: 978-1-5107-0418-3

Printed in the United States of America

I dedicate this book to Elsa Hjalmarsson Lyons, the most emphatic, generous, loving, funny, and intrinsically beautiful little sister Lina could ever wish for.

My deepest gratitude to Tony Austin Lyons, who made it possible for me to publish this book, who is the kind of father only very lucky little girls get, and without whom it would have been extremely difficult to give to both my daughters what they need. *He is a dear friend forever.*

Lilly Golden, my editor, with her sensible intelligence, fearless integrity and humor, made this book so much better and the process of working on it easy and effortless. And my appreciation and thanks go to Mike Lewis, for his patient and kind editing of the updated version/paperback.

I am also eternally grateful for my best friends, my soulsisters, Gabriella Ossoniak and Agnieszka Pawliszyn-Carmona. I can see us all on a shady porch one day when we're old and gray, animals and grandkids running in and out of the house while we are just sitting there in our comfortable rocking chairs, making jokes about our crazy lives while looking out on the vast ocean, knowing it was all good, there was nothing missing, nothing to fix or regret. . .

And Malidoma. Thank you for everything you saw and for everything you shared.

Foreword

It's not often that you hear the words "gift" and "autism" in the same sentence. Especially not when it's a struggling parent trying to make sense of this often baffling, always challenging, enigma. Yet as an autism parent myself I know the gifts of autism well—the extraordinary memory, the keen, quirky yet always insightful and piercing intelligence, the stunning lack of ego. . . .

So it was a refreshing surprise to meet Helena and immediately engage in this rare but true conversation. More refreshing yet to meet Lina, her daughter, who you will meet in this book, and see how the fruits of that unconditionally loving and accepting approach are becoming evident in the emerging brilliance of this unique young woman. Like her mother, Lina will offer something valuable to the world. Largely because of her mother.

So read this story—because Helena didn't start this way. Like most autism parents she—trying to be a good, dutiful, special needs parent—drank the Kool-Aid. The Kool-Aid of therapists and experts forcing her and the child into rigid schedules, into coercive behavioral approaches, both massively expensive and traumatic for both child and parent. The ever present pressure to put the child, or even oneself, on anti-depressants, anti-psychotics. Helena, perhaps because she is a Swede, who knows the value of the forest, of clean air, of space and room, of family and community—not to mention a good dose of Viking-inherited contempt for authority—duly flushed the Kool-Aid down the toilet and forged her own path. Humor pervades this book. You will laugh out loud. You will shed tears along with her. You will emerge at the other side refreshed and to a large degree healed, as Lina and Helena have. Follow their story, as I have, and be inspired.

—Rupert Isaacson, bestselling author of
The Horse Boy: A Memoir of Healing

Preface

To be fully, emotionally, and energetically present in life is no easy or simple feat. Finding, maintaining, and laughing at yourself, crawling on the ground, smushing rotten peaches, enduring outsiders' judgments, searching for the right home, discovering the signs of a tangible connection with your beloved daughter in the midst of spiritual tornados, revolving diets, diagnoses, and quests for hope, and mustering the strength to make it through the day without compromising your strong-willed, life-and-nature-loving, feminist beauty is a whole other level of achievement! In *Finding Lina*, we find the brutally brave and honest voice, guffawing both desperately and whimsically, of a mother, daughter, wife/ex-wife, and constant partner in parenting! We are made privy to the magic of raw love and humanity and left wanting to sip peppermint tea with this amazing mom right before she lifts up her daughters and they begin "Fire Burnin' on the Dance Floor." This book is a personal soundtrack that will accompany every mood and truth entailed in the reality of understanding and loving, unconditionally, a child with special needs and yourself along the path that is meant to be all your very own. . . . Get ready to be taken to the edge!

With great respect,
Amanda Friedman, Director,
Emerge & See Education Center

Author's Note

When I started to write this book, Lina was six years old and in the process of regaining a lot of the skills she had lost when regressing into autism around the age of three and a half. But for the last two and a half years, her development has been extremely erratic, with her being more verbal, calm, and engaged one month and with less language and more hyperactivity and meltdowns the next. One of the things I am learning to accept in being Lina's mother is that I cannot predict or control her development. The only thing I can do is be the best I can in helping her live her life the best way *she* can. This book is not so much about answers as it is about learning to find peace and joy in the face of more and more questions, increasing external challenges, and confusion. It is about trying to live in the middle of a tornado, and sometimes finding that space at the very core, where everything is still.

I have no big revelations to share about autism or any other childhood condition. I am not even sure that autism sufficiently describes what is going on with my daughter. I cannot tell you what to do when you realize that the child in your life is different. But I can share my thoughts on how I think we sometimes, in dealing with our sons and daughters or other people's special-needs children, get so ambitious in our quest to cure what we consider unacceptable that we forget to listen and be present. We get so carried away by teaching our kids to communicate in

ways that we can understand that we forget to learn to understand them. We are so busy figuring out what is going on with
our children and what to do about it, that we lose the only sure
thing we have with them, whoever they are, namely this very
moment. Of course I want a cure for Lina. And I want to do
everything in my power to help her find more words, more calm,
more ability to play, more connectedness with her old friends
and with new ones. But I also want her to feel and know deep
inside that I love her as she is, at every given moment.

This is a story about how the sudden and dramatic losses that
my daughter abruptly confronted helped me come a little closer
to an understanding of how to live my own life.

Contents

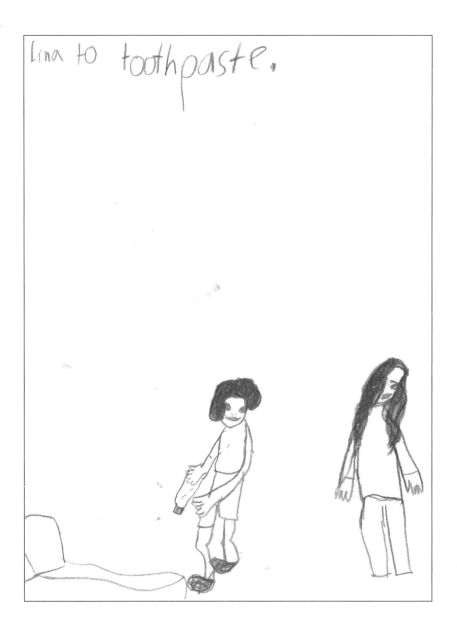

Drawing by Elsa. Lina having fun squeezing out toothpaste, while Elsa watches, bewildered.

Introduction

"Lina, NO! WAIT!"

My four-and-a-half-year-old daughter suddenly jumps up on the counter, grabs the overloaded wooden dish holder and swings it across the kitchen floor in the Newport rental house we moved into a month ago. Cups, glasses, and plates go flying and crash to the floor, transformed into a thousand pieces. Lina's beautiful face breaks out in a big devilish grin as she runs over to the art supply cabinet in the living room and, within seconds, rips out all the drawings, dumps boxes with buttons and colorful beads on the floor, finds the crayons, and starts chewing them down. Two-and-a-half-year-old Elsa, still by the table with her unfinished pancake on the plate in front of her, starts crying.

"Mama, where is my paci and my blankie?"

I run past Lina, who is still stuffing her mouth with crayons, chewing them wildly into tiny pieces and spitting them out, one by one, methodically in a circle around her on the old, wooden floor. Predictably, I find Elsa's blankie and pacifier on the futons upstairs and race back down again, three and even four steps at the time.

"Here my love, why don't you go read a few books and play a little while I help Lina to clean up."

"I want you to read for me," Elsa says and starts crying again.

"Soon, let me just take care of this," I tell her, gesturing to the shattered glass and porcelain on the floor.

I lift my chubby little friend over the shattered pieces and plop her down on the living room sofa before sprinting after Lina who has abandoned the crayons and disappeared. Running back upstairs, I find my desperately laughing daughter sitting in the bathtub, eating toothpaste.

"Lina, I know you really love that stuff but it's not good for your stomach. Here, let me put it away and we'll find something better for you to eat."

"TOOTHPASTE! TOOTHPASTE!" she shrieks with a voice that seems capable of turning our old little house into kindling. Then she throws her lean, strong body on me and bites me, hard, in the stomach. Quietly, I grab her nose, forcing her to open her mouth for air. But before I can get away, she bites again—this time much harder, right into my lower back. Screaming internally but resolved not to volunteer the reaction that would make biting even more intriguing to my confused little girl, I push toward her, trying to turn around to grab her nose again. No success. Suddenly she lets go, laughs loudly, and runs into our small bedroom, throwing herself on the two futons that cover most of the floor. I hear Elsa crying from downstairs.

"Mama, what are you doing? Come and read a book for me. What is Lina doing?" she then asks anxiously, helplessness reflected in her unsteady voice.

I shout down that I'll be there in a second, and that everything is okay. "Lina is just a little overexcited, eh?"

"Okay," she responds. I don't miss the resignation in her voice. My little two-and-a-half-year-old has been forced to accommodate what has become—impossible. I will cry later, I tell myself as I look at Lina, still in the bedroom, thrashing around on the beds. Catching a glimpse of me looking at her from the hallway, she jumps up and tries to pull down the curtains and the blinds, laughing hysterically. I walk into the tiny little room and sit down at the edge of one of the futons, making no gesture to stop Lina from completing her job.

"Lina," I say, "Lina, my love, I love you no matter what you do. No matter what."

"No matter what," Lina echoes.

"Let's go outside and swing, what do you say?"

"Swing, what do you say," she confirms.

It's one of the few things the three of us can do together apart from eating and sleeping. The large, fifty-year-old oak trees in the yard outside our house hold Lina and Elsa, now bundled in sweaters, in their swings from different branches. We sing "Swing low, sweet chariot, coming for to carry me home," and I dream away to the day when this frightening existence will be over. "A band of angels coming after me, Coming for to carry me home."

We would need a whole army of angels to carry us through this winter. A month and a half earlier, Tony and I had finally separated and moved to Newport, Rhode Island, into two separate homes. On the drive across the two bridges toward Newport, there's a tiny island located just north of Newport Bridge. There is a little shed on the island that has no windows and no doors and whoever might have lived there (no one does now) would have been exposed to water and wind, ice, and snow. To me, it became the perfect metaphor for our life that winter of 2008.

Somehow, Lina and Elsa and I managed to get through this day and many other similarly mind-boggling days. Having moved through dinner, bath, and bedtime—more food, utensils, screams, and crazed laughter flying through the air, more soap chewed on, a few big towels dumped in the bathtub water, and with biting and tearing books a predictable part of the bedtime routine, both girls, miraculously, were finally asleep. Slowly, I walked downstairs and sank down into the living room sofa, staring out onto the dark quiet street. It was February 22. My oldest brother Per had called me earlier that day from Sweden to inform me that my mother had liver cancer in its final stages. My mother had been forced to go back to Sweden earlier than expected from what would be the last of her several trips to Africa. I stared out the window for another two hours, wondering how I ended up here, with bite marks all over my arms and stomach, unable to help my daughter who sometimes reminded me more of a wild, rabies-infected animal than the lovely, affectionate little angel I once knew. How is it that things could have gotten to a point where my other little girl, only a toddler, no longer seemed to believe me when I reassured her that we were going to figure everything out? What had I been thinking moving to Newport, Rhode Island, into a house on a quiet street inhabited by cautious strangers, and, due to my little girl's rapidly progressing difficulties, unable to visit my terminally ill mother on the other side of the Atlantic?

I needed to move from the why to the how, I reminded myself as I squeezed in between Elsa and Lina—protecting the younger from the neurological unpredictability of the older.

CHAPTER ONE

Life Before Autism

I GREW UP outside of a small town in Sweden, surrounded by deep forests and lakes. Tony grew up in New York City, on the Upper West Side, surrounded by tall buildings, asphalt, noise, and people. My father was the principal of a Lutheran high school for adult students, mostly high-school dropouts getting their lives and their educations back on track. Tony's father had been an English professor, writer, and eventually a publisher, struggling with multiple jobs and long work hours to put his four children through the private Waldorf School that Tony's parents felt they ought to go to. Growing up in what at the time was one of the world's most functional socialist countries, my two older brothers and I went to public school. It wouldn't have occurred to my parents to do otherwise. Very little in my life and in my country was private. Everything in Tony's world was. My government erased the difference between rich and poor, lucky and unlucky, healthy and sick. In Tony's, you either made it or you didn't.

My mother was a temperamental choir leader and an opinionated principal's wife, a talented interior decorator and a general busybody. She was funny and charismatic, but plagued by debilitating anxiety and panic. Tony's mother is an artist. She is often quiet and introverted but her paintings are loud, large, and colorful. My parents spent long periods in Africa, both before and after my brothers and I were born, both working in a refugee camp in Sudan and within the context of a Lutheran congregation in Eritrea. I believe that my mother was drawn to Africa after her older sister had been shot there, when my mother was only a teenager. Her sister had been a dedicated missionary assistant within the Lutheran Church, and was shot by mistake by a robber who had intended to shoot the driver next to her.

Arriving in New York City in 1990, I was shocked by the inequality between people and soon found myself volunteering in soup kitchens and offering a room in my apartment to one downtrodden friend or acquaintance after another.

When Tony and I met in the summer of 1993 at a street fair we both worked at, he was fresh out of law school, studying for the bar, with large student loans and with a focused intention of securing his financial future as quickly as possible. Nothing could have been further from my mind. I worked long hours to pull together resources for graduate school, but my intention was to make the world a better place, brick by brick, step by step, person by person.

Soon, Tony flourished in publishing at a time when publishers all around him began to dip deeper and deeper into the recession. I became a privately practicing psychoanalyst. Marriage and having my own children had not been at the forefront of my life plans. Instead, I had a vision of foster kids running all around, with me and my like-minded socialist boyfriend adopting as many children as we could from broken homes. But, despite our different worldviews, Tony and I were drawn to each other. We made each other laugh, which I think is why we made it for as long as we did. And while we are both strong-willed, stubborn, and intense, humor and forgiveness still today help us find the best in each other, and to act as a team when co-parenting our daughters.

Lina was born in Connecticut. Tony had sold his and his father's book publishing company to a publisher in Connecticut, and as part of the agreement, he stayed on and worked with them for a few years. I was working as a psychotherapist in a New York City clinic and finishing up my psychoanalytic training. Westport, Connecticut, was the exact midpoint between our professional destinations.

It was a warm summer midnight in 2003, and Lina was getting ready to enter our world. Within an hour of admitting me to the hospital, Dr. Appelbee, the physician on call, came charging into the room, declaring that we needed to induce labor. One of the nurses, less temperamental than the doctor, explained to Tony and me that our baby's heart rate was dangerously low due to very low levels of amniotic fluids. Tony managed to consult a trustworthy pediatrician in New York to verify that inducing labor was necessary and things started to happen quickly.

I had planned on a natural childbirth, but now agreed to all the measures. After an epidural and a pitocin injection, I pushed Lina out in less than five minutes. There was nothing wrong with her lungs. Whenever the nurses took her into the ward to monitor her early development, her screaming rose above that of all the other babies. But she breast-fed like a champ whenever she wasn't busy screaming and passed hearing and Apgar tests with flying colors. The first night after Lina's birth the new nurse on call wanted to quiet Lina down with sugared water. I might have accepted an epidural because I was afraid of the pain but I was not about to give sugar water to my beautifully breast-feeding daughter to stop her screaming. I figured Lina had just experienced a tough trip into this new, scary life and needed to express herself. The nurse insisted that she needed to give me a break and I insisted that Tony was here should I need one. I did, reluctantly, agree to a break later that night and a proud Tony ran up and down the hallway singing "Yankee Doodle went to town, riding on a pony" to our tightly swaddled baby while carefully bouncing her. It helped. It was only our second night with our new wonderful girl and we had already figured out two powerful tricks to calm her down—breasts and Yankee Doodle, accompanied with tight wrapping and fast-paced walking, or, even better, running. This was going to be good. We congratulated each other and drove home, me in the backseat, holding the tiny hand of my fast asleep, 6.9-pound beautiful little powerhouse.

"She's pretty oral," I commented a couple of months later to my friend Carleen as we watched Lina attempting to put an entire phone in her mouth.

"That's an understatement," Carleen said.

Lina's love for exploring the world through her mouth made her a passionate breast-feeder. So passionate, in fact, that we eventually consulted a breast-feeding specialist, trying to bring down an overproduction of milk that made Lina choke, spit, cry, and scream every time she tried to feed. This same overproduction also caused my baby serious and ongoing diarrhea of the kind that made it almost impossible to prevent infected diaper rashes, which at one point, according to our stern, Harvard-educated pediatrician, only could be remedied by giving Lina antibiotics.

Before we got a handle on this dilemma, bright green liquid baby poop became a central part of our days and nights. One evening, a few months after Lina's birth, Tony and I were going to bring her with us to one of our friend's parties. Tony, dressed up in a brand new, white linen shirt, opened up Lina's diaper for the last time before we were about to jump in the car. Poop cascaded through the air and covered the entire front of Tony's shirt.

"That's it, I'm not going anywhere," he announced, trying to wipe off the green fluids from his shirt. I couldn't suppress my laughter, unaware of how one day in the not so distant future, Lina's extraordinary condition would make maintaining and developing friendships almost impossible.

Breast-feeding got back on track. Feeding repeatedly on one side before switching to the other, and letting Lina lie on top of me so as to help her not to choke on the milk, which, by the way, is called the Australian Method, brought feedings back to the blissful, connected, and restful times they had been the first month of Lina's life.

Physical closeness for Lina was essential. She slept by my side in our bed at night. During the day we wore her in a baby sling. Many mornings and late afternoons were spent walking on the nearby beach, with Lina peacefully curled up in a sling and with the sound of the gentle waves rocking her to sleep. She was always peaceful near the water. No matter how convincing her red-faced, tight-fisted, screaming agony seemed in her car seat on the short drive down to the beach, as soon as we opened the doors to let the air and the wind and the sound of the water register, she always shifted, becoming the most easygoing little baby-Buddha anyone had ever seen. So we spent increasing time down there, at the beach. Water was clearly her element. Whether at the beach or in a little plastic bassinet that served as her bathtub the first six months of her life, Lina was always in a good mood.

During most of Lina's waking hours, I worked actively to elicit smiles and sounds from her. Every day I invented new games to catch her attention. Being that Lina was my first, I had no sense of this being an unusually intense motherly approach. Sometimes, relatives and friends might try to point something out about the universe outside of Lina, but such comments only registered in the periphery. Instinctively, I must have known that Lina needed every extra hour of active engagement. But it was not a conscious choice. Not something I hesitated to do or resolved to commit to. Never something someone recommended. It was the way I was a mother to Lina. I thought it was similar to the way everyone mothered their babies and children. Only later, as I participated in a group of Swedish mothers, did I realize that I was pretty much the only one doing this. If I modified my involvement with Lina, played a little less with her, let her be by herself for a few minutes, she either fell apart, screamed, or seemed . . . absent. One day I decided to put Lina in the stroller instead of the sling and go for a long walk to a nearby park. We were about an hour away from home when Lina suddenly turned from cheerful to screaming. It was the kind of howling that instantly became the center of attention for everyone in the park, including a tall, slim man with his long hair in a ponytail, who stood on top of a little hill, worshipping the sun. With a poorly diffused edge, he demanded to know if I had fed my screaming girl and if she was cold. With equal irritation, I responded that I had indeed fed her and being that it was the middle of a warm summer day, I wasn't too concerned about my daughter being cold. The man forgot the sun, pointed his long, skinny finger at me, and shouted, "IT IS YOU! IT IS YOU! THAT'S THE PROBLEM! SHE IS SCREAMING BECAUSE OF YOUUU!!"

We eventually got home. And as soon as we did, Lina calmed down. In fact, most of the time, as long as I stayed right beside her, shared my substantial milk supply (it would have been enough to feed at least ten other babies) without reserve, and had her in a sling for a couple of hours each day, she was happy and developed beautifully. The sling was useful not only to me but also to Tony.

Lina and I were rarely apart. Keeping up a part-time psychoanalytic practice did require that I spend a couple of half days in the city. Sweetly and generously, Tony drove us all into the city those days and delivered Lina to me in between my sessions so that we could be together and Lina could breast-feed. Frequently, we all stayed over in a hotel and loved being in the city again. In the hotel room, Lina discovered the bathtub for the first time, since the apartment that we rented in Westport only had a shower. She would splash around in the bathtub smiling broadly, needing a lot of cajoling to let herself be picked up and wrapped in the plush hotel bath towels. And I loved not having to worry about cleaning and cooking, and using up as many towels as we wanted. And Tony, most of all, loved spending time back on the streets of New York City. When Lina was six months old, this arrangement turned into permanent living, and we moved back to the Upper West Side where both of us had lived for most of our adult lives. Tony was able to spend increasing time working from home, and I started to see my clients from home. It was such a relief to be back in the city. We had beautiful Central Park two blocks away from us, as well as Riverside Park, with its lovely Boat Basin, trails along the water, and multiple play-grounds, a block west of our bright, charming, high-ceilinged apartment. And Lina continued developing beautifully, babbling and playing, laughing and giggling, and being so connected and aware of everything and everyone around her.

Soon after we were back in the city, I met a mother who became one of my closest friends. Her daughter was the same age as Lina and soon turned into my daughter's most impor-tant friend. Ellen. Little precocious, lovely, brown-eyed Ellen. A teacher from the start, just like her mother. Ellen had her hands full with Lina, who always did what she believed made sense and what she wanted to do rather than following some-body else's rules, who was probably the most self-directed little friend Ellen would ever come across. Lina and Ellen became inseparable. We started them at the same preschool, and parents of other children in their class frequently expressed insecurity about their own children's level of interactivity compared to the evolved and interactive play they witnessed between Ellen and Lina. Ellen's mother, my dear friend Anki, and her husband

Anders moved from the Lower East Side into our building. All of a sudden we had a community! Biweekly dinners, shared Christmases and vacations, endless playdates, coffee breaks, and dropping each other's children off in our respective apartments all became part of our lives. Celebrating life became our daily mission and no one was more skilled at creating festivities and celebration than Anki. Everyone around her felt happy. I have, in most instances, had a kind of clarity about whom I wanted very close to me. A kind of inborn bullshit detector that helps me trust what I see beyond people's verbal presentation of themselves. Listening to Anki, I did see some fear, some internalized social pressure, someone who has frequently been cornered into the role of a mediator. But I also saw so much love and light and goodwill that laughing and smiling and kidding around naturally became part of what I did in Anki's company. I used to joke that if we both hadn't been married, and I had been a man, or, alternatively, a lesbian, I would have proposed to Anki. She was so easy to be around. With the growing tension in Tony's and my relationship, spending time with Anki felt like a relief, a kind of protection from being sucked into what was beginning to feel like a dark hole. Tony and I found it increasingly difficult to laugh at our disagreements and help each other through difficult times. But when Anki and I had rough times with the kids, we supported each other and when that didn't help we just laughed it off.

And when our daughter Elsa came into the world, Tony and I went off to Cornell Medical Center in a cab across Central Park, while Anki, with her big belly ready to give birth any moment herself, slept faithfully next to Lina. She comforted my daughter when she woke up in the middle of the night crying for me and gently stroked her back until she fell back to sleep. There was no one I would rather have there with Lina that night than this friend. I felt so lucky. When Anki's little warrior, Alfred, with lung capacity similar to Lina's, was born, I rocked Ellen to sleep in my arms and woke her up to a pancake breakfast with her best friend Lina. I have a picture of the two of them, sitting side by side in the bright red double stroller we had just bought, sleepy-eyed and serious, waiting for pancakes to be ready and for Ellen's new brother to arrive home from the hospital.

Lina was thriving and seemed to adjust generously to Elsa. Our little two-year-old sat around with Elsa proudly in her lap and handed Elsa all of her own most precious possessions—her favorite dolls, the plastic pieces of food that she loved to play with, big chunks of Play-Doh, the plastic cube that produced Mozart and Vivaldi music as well as the sounds of individual instruments when you pressed on the different sides. She even let her little sister sniffle on the most valued possession, her blankie. Lina showed an unusually generous, non-possessive personality that protected her from being caught in ways that many people are caught, in defensiveness, fear, and inability to let go.

Elsa, in turn, was the easiest baby I had ever met. From the morning of her birth, in hot August of 2005, Elsa has seemed to accept everything in her life almost effortlessly. I can't bank on that, I remind myself, and only barely manage to avoid psychoanalyzing Elsa as the already parentified child, needing so much less attention and holding than her sister; in comparison seeming almost unnaturally self-sufficient, as if she already subconsciously knew that there was only room for one high maintenance child in the family. She wasn't, of course. Not at that time. Because at that point life didn't seem any more challenging for us than for any other family with a couple of small children. It was busy but we had a rich, fun-filled life with two gorgeous, interesting little girls making it even more wonderful.

With much support, encouragement, and inspiration from her older sister, Elsa grew up to be an imaginative toddler. She often stunned us with stories that were rich and innovative, intelligent and emphatic. Today, it is hard to remember that Lina, at two and a half, could have been Elsa's most mutual and interactive playmate. As a toddler, Lina was that imaginative and verbally expressive child. She happily played with Ellen and Elsa and anyone else, big or small, who came through our doors for a visit. Watching old videos, I see her standing by the toy stove in our 81st Street apartment, located just off Broadway. Ellen is on the other side of the stove. Both girls are cooking busily. Elsa sits in a rhythmically moving child seat, watching it all.

"Mama," Lina says in Swedish, "I'm done with the cooking."

"You're done?" I respond, also in Swedish. "What did you make? It looks like . . . what is that, peas?"

Lina pauses and gives me a concentrated, inquisitive look.

"No, no, no," she laughs, pointing at the video camera, asking, "that's a . . ."

"It's a video camera. And what do you have? Is it a pancake?"

"No!" she shouts as she skips back to the stove, picks up some plastic salad and, triumphantly, informs me: "Broccolella!" She gives this freshly invented vegetable to me and rushes back to the stove.

Lina starts singing: "Macalola, Macalola." Ellen responds: "Macalola, Macalola." Lina goes back over to where I'm sitting next to Elsa. Elsa makes a throaty sound. "Ahhhhgaaa."

"Tomato, Elsa, that's tomato, Elsa," Lina says, switching from Swedish to English as she gives the tomato piece to her little sister.

"Mmm, tomato for Elsa, so good," I affirm.

"Oh, no," huffs Ellen, still in English, picks up a pretend French fry from the floor. Lina goes back to the stove to work on the next scenario.

"You will not have that anymore," Lina says, puts the cheese in the sink, walks back to me, and says firmly: "You will not have cheese anymore."

"No?" I ask, acting concerned, "Isn't there any more cheese?"

"No more," Lina states, matter-of-factly.

"No?" I repeat, increasing my concern slightly, and stare at Lina. She breaks out smiling. Her face beams with compassion mixed with a wonderful, humorous glimpse.

"Mama, mama, you *can* have cheese."

"Oh, thank you, my friend, thank you, my love, I was getting a bit worried. Mmmm, it's so good."

"So we can eat cheese!" Lina concludes, as she clasps her hands together in a hospitable, celebratory way.

Lina's nurturing, generous style defined her personality. She fed, medicated, sang for, entertained, hugged, and kissed everyone around her. This, in spite of (or maybe partly because of) the fact that I had to abruptly end Lina's access to my breast milk when she was eighteen months old, shortly before Elsa's birth, due to contractions that threatened to cause premature labor. Only once, Lina explicitly protested me giving Elsa the milk that just recently had been Lina's most precious source of nutrition and comfort.

Lina did experience the losses involved in getting a little baby sister. Tony and I had talked a lot about how to make the transition from being an only child to a sibling of a tiny, needy baby as smooth as possible. Maybe because Tony sometimes had experienced feeling like the third wheel in the context of Lina's and my relationship, he was particularly concerned that Lina now would suffer. One night after Lina went to sleep Tony showed me a letter that he had written right before Elsa's birth to Dr. William Sears, a well-known pediatrician who is particularly knowledgeable about breast-feeding issues.

"Dear Dr. Sears," Tony wrote, "we have an eighteen-month-old child who is very attached to her mother. They sleep together, talk Swedish together (I'm American), breast feed together (twice a day—before the nap and night sleep) and have an intensely close relationship (though I spend a lot of time with our daughter, too). We're soon going to have a second baby and we're concerned that the strong attachment between mother and daughter might make the transition difficult for our daughter and us."

Dr. Sears never responded to Tony's letter. But reading it helped me understand my husband better. He was not just describing Lina's potential challenges, but also his own, potential as well as already actualized. And Lina, well, she mostly enjoyed Elsa and, with impressive instinct, weaved her into her games. Most of the time, she seemed so ready to have a little sibling. Never did Lina try to exclude Elsa when other people were around. She always just assigned different roles and functions to Elsa and skillfully welcomed her little sister into her rich social network.

CHAPTER TWO

Searching for Home

Life had been so good this year, with our best friends upstairs and with Lina and Elsa becoming such interesting little people. Tony and I didn't do nearly as well as our daughters. We have, and always have had, so much love between us. Neither Tony nor I hold onto negative things, which, paradoxically, might have been the factor causing us to hold onto our marriage a little too long. This is not a story about Tony and me. Of course our difficulties influenced both Lina and Elsa. The increasing frequency of difficult days. The unpredictability of our lives together. For the most part, no one screamed, but anger and sadness became part of our lives. Our apartment building was sold. Tony and I moved to an apartment on 86th Street that had belonged to the deceased father of a friend. Lina and I, in particular, missed the comfort of our upstairs friends. When Lina approached her third year, I felt myself slipping into a depression that somehow prevented me from making good decisions. I knew at this time that Tony and I needed time apart. My close friends knew. Most likely, Tony's close friends were equally convinced. Even Lina knew. In the context of an argument between Tony and me, Lina looked me in the eyes and sadly commented, "A building is falling down on Mama."

Then, in November of 2006, when Lina was three and a half years old, something happened to her—she left us in a way that terrified all of us. She had been with Therese, our wonderful, Swedish babysitter, in Riverside Park. Lina, sitting on the swing, suddenly seemed out of it. She hadn't responded when Therese called her name. She had just stared right through her, as if she didn't know that Therese was there. Therese took her home. Lina was okay for the rest of that day. The next day and the day after, she would start to cry for no apparent reason. She seemed phobic and would often run after me, suddenly, as if something had just terrorized her internally and she needed my protection.

One of those frightening days, Anki and Ellen were coming by our apartment. It was Wednesday and even though we were living in different buildings at this point, we stayed faithful to our weekly Wednesday tradition of having dinner at each other's houses. But this day was very different. Saliva began to flow out of Lina's mouth and she stared at me, expressionless.

"Lina," I begged her, feeling seconds away from panic, "please swallow. Can't you just swallow? Please, Lina."

Anki looked at me, mirroring my own sense of desperation. Right then, in that moment, trying in vain to convince my strangely unavailable daughter to swallow, I caught the first glimpse of the indescribable nightmare that would become such a predictable part of my everyday life. I didn't know then that the time would come when my daughter would not be able to do other things we took for granted: to speak, look me in the eyes, play with toys, stop herself from pushing and hitting her little sister or biting me until no part of my arms and stomach was without that familiar blue-and-green-colored pattern of little, sharp teeth. That afternoon, Lina received a referral from our pediatrician to see a specialist at the New York Medical Center for Epilepsy.

At dinnertime that night, the food that Lina put in her mouth fell out as she was unable to control her jaw muscles. Tony and I looked at each other. Fear and agony united us. That night, Tony expressed his fear that our marital difficulties were responsible for Lina's breakdown. He blamed himself. I watched him sit down on the couch. He looked broken. Scared by the sound of my own words, I told him that I thought this might be something beyond what had transpired between him and me. "We will know more after the appointment," I told my crushed husband. "Let's hold off with blame and conclusions. We will continue to do the best we can." I hugged Tony on the couch and told him I loved him and walked down the hallway to my daughters' bedroom. I lay down next to Lina, praying that whatever it was that had created that terrifying, vacant look in her face would be gone in the morning.

It wasn't. Lina still said almost nothing. Drool kept flowing down her sagging chin. It had only been two weeks since Lina had endured her second MMR shot. But neither Tony nor I, nor anyone else around us, suspected that this grueling experience had anything to do with the vaccination. Instead of taking her to school, I placed her in the child seat at the back of my orange mountain bike and brought her across town to the NYU Medical Center where we were to meet Dr. LaJoise, specialist in childhood epilepsy. Lina didn't say much as we entered the lobby of the center. She just held my hand tightly, unsure of what was going to happen next. By then she was able to eat and hold the food a little better in her mouth but as soon as she stopped chewing, drool would begin to drop out of her mouth again.

Dr. LaJoise explained what was about to happen. The doctor was an attractive, petite, African American woman whose gracious, respectful demeanor and careful explanations made me instantly trust her. She wanted Lina to have a twenty-minute electroencephalogram (EEG), a test to measure brain electrical activity, before meeting with us to gather information. Lina was very accepting of the not-so-pleasant and, for her, quite incomprehensible procedure of the EEG with strange little colorful cords taped all around her head. But as long as I stayed right next to her, held her hand, looked into her beautiful big eyes, and sang songs for her, she was content. As long as she was able to be near me, and be held, hugged, and sung to, she was happy. I felt so grateful for the bond between us that would help her through this traumatic, unexpected hurdle. The discussion with Dr. LaJoise following the EEG turned into a mutual brainstorming of underlying causes of this mysterious drooling episode.

While ordering an extended EEG, the doctor seemed reluctant to suspect epilepsy and more inclined to consider the possibility that Lina displayed a temporary regression caused either by some sort of infection or, possibly, by stressors of a failing marriage, a new sibling, a new school, and a move from one apartment to another. I decided to wait and see before putting Lina through the experience of an extended EEG. As we biked home, Lina, who hadn't napped for the past year, fell asleep in the seat behind me. I looked back at her, feeling the honor of being responsible for the well-being of this little, wonderful, interesting, and unusual human being. Since then, this feeling of awe, the experience of being asked to do something beyond my own ability, something sacred, has never left me. My heart filled with determined love. I believe every mother who has ever experienced their child as truly vulnerable understands this.

Just a few days after this appointment, results from Lina's pediatrician's blood test showed that Lina had Epstein-Barr virus. For two long weeks, Lina had recurring moments of seeming out of it and confused.

Walking across Central Park on the way to a fall fair arranged by the Rudolf Steiner School, where Lina had started a couple of months prior, Lina intermittently said, "Where is our street?," "Can I eat that one?," and "Hello, mama," over and over again. Back home again, she became upset and cried every time I left the room. I soon abandoned the idea of this regression being due to environmental or emotional stress. When I think of autism, I think about it as the perfect storm of a whole array of factors coinciding in a child's life and making her vulnerable to a kind of neurological breakdown. The severity of Lina's symptoms and the dramatic onset pointed to a neurological confusion and disarray likely caused by the MMR shot and the subsequent Epstein-Barr virus. Two weeks later, all signs of drooling were gone. Gradually, Lina returned to her usual cheerful, interactive self. There was no end to the relief and gratefulness Tony and I felt about this recovery.

That fall, Lina's new teacher had noticed how our daughter seemed to take a long time to get involved with the other kids and often spent time by herself. During their class's daily walk and free-play time in Central Park, Lina sometimes walked off, beyond the boundaries set by the teachers. Lina's teacher also commented on how Lina's grip, as she was holding the teacher's hand, seemed less firm than other children's. While the idea of Lina's less firm hand-holding confused me, my daughter's teacher and I discussed ideas about how we could support Lina's greater involvement with her friends. Typically the Rudolf Steiner School discourages parents with new students from arranging playdates between the children in their class. It was important for the group to form as a whole and playdates between certain kids would prevent that from happening. Now, however, Lina's teacher thought I should arrange playdates with the children in the class. I did. After school, Lina hung out with Malina, Violet, Jonas, and Ethan. She quickly began to become a more integral part of the group. Her use of language and pretend play, which seemed to have stagnated in school that fall and even, to a much lesser extent, at home, again began to flourish. She developed another close friendship, with a girl who eventually moved back to Israel where her family had come from. Her name was Mika. Both Tony and I became close friends with Mika's parents, Orit and Ynon. Her mother is sweetness, sincerity, and good-heartedness embodied. Her father has a much more low-key charm and a calm and quiet warmth and friendliness. Mika seemed the perfect combination of her parents. Lina loved Mika. They were twin souls. With the exception of Ellen, I have never seen Lina more comfortable and connected with another child.

Nothing was more reassuring to me when I worried about Lina's social development than to see her run around with Mika in the wooded areas of Riverside or Central Park—getting dirty, collecting stones or bugs or sticks, and running after each other shouting and laughing about things that were incomprehensible to the outsider. They gave each other space. Every time they were together, each was intuitively respectful of the other's need to warm up slowly to the interaction. No one was the leader. No one dominated. It was pure magic between two people. Watching them together was better than watching the perfect love affair.

Part of being a parent to a child with special needs is the endless retrospective attempts to trace my own initial awareness of something being wrong. This, of course, is partly to figure out if I could have done something sooner, if I missed something that could have changed my child's future. It is the agonizing thought process about whether it was, in fact, my own fault in some way that Lina developed autism. Such thoughts, as long as we are overpowered by our own minds, are inevitable and I don't believe the parents of a child with autism exist who haven't, at some point, asked themselves, "What did we do wrong?" Soon after Ynon, Orit, and Mika moved back to Israel, I wrote the following to Orit:

> *Lina seems to be doing well at Rudolf Steiner though she sometimes says it's "no fun" and she doesn't want to go. Hard to gauge whether it's just her regular transition difficulties or something else. . . . Don't know what it is with me lately but I find myself worrying so much about Lina. Tony tells me to stop but I don't seem to be able to. I might confuse myself with her or I might be onto something but how does one know the difference?*

Eventually, my worries subsided somewhat. Lina seemed to return to her usual expressive, charismatic, and quirky self. That spring, Tony and I felt sure that whatever the cause of the difficulties during the fall, Lina, approaching her fourth birthday, had conquered them and was back to her normal and present self. Love, I figured, will heal Lina.

In the aftermath of Lina's intense regression, Tony and I continued to try to patch up our relationship. Our transition from being a couple to becoming a family with two children was not going so well. Tony felt that I gave our daughters every ounce of energy and warmth I had, not leaving enough for him. He felt abandoned and lonely. His ambition to understand and define our relationship kept my engagement with him alive. But despite these efforts we felt ourselves slipping away from each other.

Our search for a better way of relating to each other went on for years. We disagreed on all kinds of things. One was child care. Tony wanted more help from babysitters. I wanted less. But his point that "any time one of us is sick or tired or anything, our marriage falls apart" was well taken. We didn't have endless stamina.

So, we hired Marion, one of Lina's preschool teachers. She welcomed opportunities for extra work and started coming to take care of the girls on Friday nights. And it was wonderful just to leave the house and go outside without the kids. It gave us time to walk together and talk. Sometimes we argued about where to live. Moving or not moving circulated around what would be best for Lina. She loved smaller contexts, familiar people, few crowds, more social safety and predictability than the life that New York City offered. She loved hills and trees to climb, soil to dig in, water to splash in. I had brought the girls to Sweden for a couple of weeks while Tony stayed in New York to work. Both Lina and Elsa loved the small town, being surrounded by relatives, the easy access to lakes and trees.

Tony voted for Westport, where Lina had been born. But Westport, with its wealthy, materialistic, suburban residents worried me. We had found our niche and good friends when we had lived there three years earlier. But going back as a family, and having our children become absorbed into the public school system there, didn't seem ideal either. I leaned toward Rhode Island, but it would have been too far of a commute to New York City, where I still had my part-time practice and Tony now ran a new publishing venture.

Lacking a perfect solution, we moved back to Westport, hoping that it would be a simpler life with better opportunities for long-term friendships for our daughters (Lina had already lost Mika when they moved back to Israel and was about to lose her very best friend, Ellen, whose family had plans to move back to Sweden the following year.) We wanted to give our girls proximity to trees, water, and open spaces. We hoped to have more time to be with our girls without the financial pressure of New York City life. We wished for both of them to have a back-yard and plenty of opportunity to run around freely, without having to be strapped into a stroller or constantly having to hold someone's hand. The name Lina is a short derivative of Karolina, the female version of Karl, which has Germanic origins and means "free man." From very early on, Lina has always struck me as an unusually freedom-hungry child. She needed to eat, sleep, play, and talk in her own way. Knowing that neither Lina nor I would benefit, I avoided engaging in power struggles with her unless absolutely necessary. We found our own ways to negotiate. Trust developed. She trusted me. When I really needed her to do something—go to the doctor with me, wait for Elsa to breast-feed before I could hold her at night before sleeping, kiss her friend and apologize for snatching her food—she usually did as I asked. I trusted her. If she really felt that she needed to go outside to run around, climb on something, swing on something, or just be near some trees or water, I would try my damnedest to accommodate her. If she felt she really needed a certain kind of food, as long as it was relatively healthy, I tried to get it for her. Later on, we learned about all the benefits of various diets, including gluten- and dairy-free ones. But at this point, Lina still didn't have a diagnosis, and was still doing okay with eating healthy, wholesome, mostly organic foods.

Moving to Westport could have been great. We could have arranged for beautiful family nature trips every weekend and had our backyard filled with friends and friends' children almost every day. I could have started to establish myself as a psycho-analyst out there and Tony could have spent a lot of his work week at home or even moved his company to some nearby town, maintaining the closeness with his growing children and with me. But instead, we failed, miserably.

Everything started to fall apart—our marriage, Lina, our social life—which affected Lina and Elsa the most and life as we all imagined it. Maybe it had something to do with our worries about Lina, who began to have more difficulties making connections with new friends and seemed to be in constant motion. Maybe it was the fact that the friends we had made when we'd last lived in Westport had all moved away and now we were suddenly surrounded by the real Westporters, almost exclusively white and affluent. I don't know, but I do remember looking out the window of the house we rented, seeing Mexican workers coming in with little trucks to mow some of our rich neighbors' lawns, and wondering about the soundness of my decision-making ability. This was a different Westport than I remembered from last time we lived there, when we had our house filled with Lithuanian friends, playing Ping-Pong until everyone dripped with sweat and the old, wooden house was shaking with laughter. Now, we met parents at the beach who passionately argued for keeping special-needs children out of regular schools. This was before Tony and I had any idea that Lina would be one of the kids that they wanted to keep out. But the thought was no less alienating. I didn't remember neighbors like the couple next door who withdrew their kind good-mornings because of a fence that we put up to keep our little freedom-hungry Lina safe, right after she had slipped out of the house while I was putting Elsa down for a nap.

In this way and others, Lina's specialness gradually became more apparent. Teachers at her new school, Earth Place—characterized by the very thing that Lina was good at, nature excursions and wildlife—complained that Lina was too much of an excursioner. They also noted that she had walked on top of the science table one day and that another day, she had eaten the uncooked rice from the sensory corner. She spoke less often, particularly at school. And her language became less direct and less personal. More and more of her communication was focused on requests rather than expressing things about herself and her environment. She didn't connect as effectively with her classmates as other children did. She didn't find a best friend like she had in the past. While Lina did much better at home than in school, she seemed quieter, less joyful and increasingly restless and hyperactive even at home. My sense of alarm became a permanent knot in my stomach. Betsy, an early childhood consultant, observed Lina in school and noted Lina's sensory-seeking behavior.

"She is such a beautiful, cheerful, and affectionate child, but she is not participating as much as the other children," she told me after her visit to the school. "She seems to crave sensory input, always putting all kinds of things in her mouth, always moving around, distracted and searching for sensory experience." It was true. Lina did not just try to put everything in sight in her mouth, but she would also lean against large objects, press herself against the bodies of people she knew in whatever way they let her, climb everything in sight, seemed to enjoy being out in powerful winds or pouring rain, and loved snow and ice. Betsy recommended that I read *The Out of Sync Child* by Carol Stock Kranowitz. I did and was relieved. Lina embodied the out of sync child. She seemed to fit the criteria for Sensory Processing Disorder with her constant mouthing, her increasing need for constant motion, her excessive need to be held, bounced, rocked, pressed against. As explained in *The Out of Sync Child*, Lina's overwhelming need for a wide variety of sensory input distracted her from important developmental learning. She often seemed too preoccupied with putting food and toys in her mouth to be able to concentrate on connecting with a neighbor's girl, who was four and a half years old, just a few months older than Lina, and dying to have a playmate on her street. Instead, Lina began talking to herself. Sometimes what she said made sense, and other times Lina's self-talk didn't make much sense at all. The days when Lina had walked around in our New York City apartment, musing over what her little sister was doing, now seemed like the distant past.

"But what is Elsa doing?" she had wondered playfully.

"I don't know," I would say. "What are *you* up to?"

Lina would shrug and make a little twirling dance around Elsa, laughing and singing for her young admirer and for me and anyone else who was around. This charismatic showing off was rare now. She no longer invented imaginary people to have pretend phone conversations with. She frequently climbed on furniture and windowsills. She would climb on the staircase railing in our Westport house a hundred times a day. She talked less and less, and often seemed not to hear or pay attention to what people around her were saying. She was restless and constantly on the move. The unauthorized excursions that her teachers had complained about became noticeable at home with me as well. One day, I was coming downstairs to the sun-filled living room to have some special time with Lina after putting Elsa down for a nap. Lina was not on the couch where she usually waited for me, looking forward to time shared by just me and her as much as I did. She wasn't in the kitchen or in the bathroom. Trying to push away the bad feeling in my gut, I ran upstairs, three, four steps at a time, checking Tony's office, the guest room. As I ran from room to room still without a sight of Lina I cursed at the big house, hiding my daughter. But it was an unfair accusation. Lina wasn't in it. I quickly checked on Elsa, observing her calm breathing, and ran downstairs again, out of the goddamn house, out onto the street. She was nowhere. An eternal minute later I heard myself screaming Lina's name as I sprinted toward the busy street in front of our house leading toward the beach. A very fast hundred yards later I saw a police car parked outside one of the larger houses on the road. A woman with bleached hair and an unfriendly smirk on her face, a neighbor to whom I had never spoken and had hardly ever seen, stood next to the police car with Lina's hand firmly in hers. I ran up to Lina, throwing my arms around her, tears instantly pouring down my face.

"Oh, baby, please, my little friend, wait for me next time, will you?" Lina looked at me, melting into my arms. But when I looked into her eyes I had to wonder, did she understand the seriousness of this? Would she wait for me next time? Or would she once again be driven away from me and from safety by some unknown force much stronger than my protective love?

"You better look out for her next time, not just letting her run around without anybody looking after her," the indignant neighbor said, as if reading my own thoughts about what was happening to Lina. I looked at her, then at Lina, resisting the urge to lash out at the opinionated neighbor, took Lina by the hand, and quietly thanked the woman for holding on to her.

That weekend, we put up a fence in the backyard.

At the time, that fence was the only thing I truly liked about the monstrous rental house we were living in. Our next-door neighbors, an older, miserable couple who screamed at each other for long hours every other night, disliked it immensely. One day after the new fence construction, which quite possibly could save Lina from injuries and even premature death, the lady of the house lectured me about the responsibility we all had toward each other in preserving the market value of the estates in the area by *not* doing things like building distasteful fences in our yards. Her point was that this is a way that we are all connected to each other. She felt that we all had to cultivate a sense of respect and commonality. I had been wondering about that. How does one connect with one's neighbors in a neighborhood like this? Especially someone like me, who grew up in a country with the most successfully implemented socialism the world has ever seen. I began to suspect that I was going to have to take my girls out of this neighborhood. I wanted to raise them in a community where people understand that what happens to your neighbor, happens to you. I had an uneasy feeling that God must be quite amused at the sight of his little feminist rebel, misplaced in a neighborhood where people care more about materialistic prestige and real estate value than keeping young citizens safe. I wasn't able to be accepting of what I saw around me. I judged people right and left. And I judged myself, for being part of it all.

"I'm sorry you're unhappy about the fence. If it's any comfort to you, we probably won't live here for very long," I responded, struggling to keep easily accessible insults and curse words from escaping my lips.

"I'm really not sure if we'll be able to allow this."

I snapped, informing her that for however long we did live there, the fence would stay where it was, and spun away, as scornful of this woman's greed as she was of my fence.

"Your mother is very nice," this same lady neighbor said one day after one of my mother's rare visits to the United States, giving me her first genuine smile since we'd moved in there.

"Uhum," I said, with something between a smile and a grimace.

"Very charming and lovely in every way." My neighbor looked at me with some level of reconciliation, but also seemed to sincerely wonder how a lovely woman such as my mother could possibly be dealt an offspring like the tough person in braids and torn shorts, who danced to loud hip-hop music with her unruly daughters, standing in front of her.

Equally confused, instead of accepting her experience of my mother as it was, I silently wondered, "How is it that my mother, who cannot, by any stretch of the imagination, be described as motherly, have produced someone who makes a happy living out of helping people become happy and calm and who loves nothing better than being with and providing for her daughters, and yet has a child who runs away from home?" For me, at this point, God was someone to negotiate with rather than an internal wisdom and resource. "God," I half prayed, half argued, "I'm not really ready to talk to you yet, but you should know that sometimes I don't get you or your master plan."

A few months later, after only half a year in Connecticut, we packed up again. We were moving to Newport, Rhode Island, to the real ocean, to an island with nature preserves, bird sanctuaries, apple and strawberry picking, and fresh air. We were hoping to build a community, fostering an exchange between families with different backgrounds, taking care of each others' children, have a horse in our backyard and eventually grow our own vegetables together. Our long-time friends Michael and Lauren with their four children were the starting point. We were hoping that Lina, who thrives in reoccurring, predictable social situations with familiar people, who is a nature child, who loves the ocean and bodysurfing on the waves, would get back to her normal self and start talking and listening and responding and relating again. Elsa, well, Elsa would thrive anywhere. In retrospect I realize that the constant moving and changing our external conditions represented our difficulties facing our own pain. As long as we kept focusing on our external conditions, not much would change on the inside. But I didn't know that then.

CHAPTER THREE

Disillusion

Tony and I moved into different houses. Mine was in the middle of a quiet street next to a playground. It had a lovely little backyard with an old oak tree. The large tree had sturdy, thick branches that Lina and Elsa could pretend were the backs of horses. Soon, those same branches held two swings and a climbing ladder, and the girls loved it. The old wooden house preserved light and warmth in the winter like a bear in hibernation. In the summer, the old oak in the backyard provided much-needed shade and the house, miraculously, stayed cool without air conditioners or even fans. Tony's house was on the other side of the playground, a five-minute walk from mine. There was no tree in Tony's garden but he had an attic with incredible light and with brand new, off-white, very soft and inviting wall-to-wall carpet. Before the move, Tony and I had kept our explanation of the separation to the kids optimistic and simple. "When we get to Newport," we told them, "Mama and Papa are going to live in different houses. You will stay mostly with Mama but when Mama is working you'll get to stay with Papa. We have figured out that we'll get along better that way. And we think that will be better for everyone. We both love you two so much."

The first months after our separation, the getting along part wasn't too impressive. But with Tony still working in New York City and me going in for Friday afternoons and Saturday morning appointments, we did get the much needed space that helped us reformulate ourselves from married, together, and disappointing each other, to separate, alone, responsible and free to create our own lives with the girls in whatever way we thought best. Had it not been for Lina's neurological challenges (we still didn't label it autism though the thought began to lurk in the back of our minds), life in Newport might have been different. The first glaring shift from hope to disillusion came about the very first day there. Our friends Michael and Lauren had generously offered for us to stay at their house the first couple of days so that both Tony and I could make our houses ready for Lina and Elsa. Lina, restless and uprooted, and sensory-seeking as usual, got into everything in Michael and Lauren's house. It being the week before Christmas, she found wrapped Christmas presents on one of her scavenger hunts. Being Lina, she unwrapped the presents and checked them out before anyone had time to stop her. The next morning, Lauren approached me as I quickly gulped down some coffee before running out of the house to get to work on making my new house as welcoming and familiar as possible for the girls.

"Helena, I would prefer it if you brought the girls with you instead of leaving them here," she said.

I stared at Lauren, thinking I must have somehow misunderstood what I just had heard, since Sarah, our babysitter, would be staying to take care of Lina and Elsa. But when I explained this, Lauren said, "Well, actually, even if Sarah is with them, I would rather that you take them with you. Lina got into the presents yesterday and she is eating everything in sight, food or not food, and quite frankly it's not so easy for Sarah to catch her. I just don't feel like dealing with wrapping those presents again. So I would really appreciate it if you just brought the girls with you."

I looked at Lauren. She was serious. No question. But for the sake of my precious jewels I was willing to live with injured pride and make one more attempt to make her understand. I didn't know then that this was to become how most people would react to Lina's behavior. My own experience was still so incomprehensible and intense, there simply was no room to take in and understand much about anybody else's. My girls had been through so many changes. I just wanted them to be able to enter their new home with some of their familiar things in place. I also knew that unpacking would be next to impossible with Lina around.

"Lauren, I'm just going to run over there to fix up the bedroom and make it a little more inviting for the girls, okay? I'll be right back."

She reluctantly agreed. I ran over to my house and sprinted from room to room in a panic, trying to pull out some of the most deeply loved toys from boxes and set up the bedroom as sweat poured down my face. *It's okay,* I said to myself, *Everything will be okay. This is a great house and it'll be a splendid home for my lovely girls and we'll have peace. We have a new chance....* Just as I was pep-talking myself, Michael came in, smiling broadly. "Wow, you're fast. It's beginning to look like someone lives here. What can I do?"

I don't remember much of the girls' reaction to our new home. I do know that the weeks after Christmas and the month January of 2008 were ... rough. Somehow, I got it in my head that a good school for Lina would be a big part of the solution. Our plans were to put Lina in a Montessori school run by Lauren's sister. No formal interviews were necessary. Lina would be welcome to start as soon as we were settled in and ready. A week after our Newport arrival, Lina and I visited the school. My little four-and-a-half-year-old was restless and distracted. As we sat down briefly to join the other kids for circle time, I noticed a slowly expanding dark circle on the wall-to-wall carpet around Lina. Being toilet-trained was one aspect of Lina's development that had regressed after what we all now recognized had been a seizure the year before. She had improved since then, but over the past couple months, with increasing frequency, Lina had begun to have accidents. It wasn't that she had anything in particular against the toilet; she would use it often—but her success at making it in time had become hit or miss. The orientation session ended in frenzy with me leaving Lina in the bathroom, running to the car to rummage around for something for her to wear, and with Montessori teachers running in and out of the playroom with wet towels to mop up the carpet. I thought I had prepared the school for Lina's increasingly unusual behavior, but after a few days I received a letter from Lauren's sister stating that they were in no position to accept Lina into their school. Their view was that Lina was a special-needs child and that they weren't equipped to handle such children at their school. She ended the letter by listing some names of people and organizations who might be able to help. There it was in writing. We could no longer ignore the fact that Lina was special.

At the same time as I was looking for a new school, I started the evaluation process for Lina. Her new pediatrician recommended neurologist William Brown in nearby Providence. Lina smiled happily for Dr. Brown as she skipped into the examination room, seeming to experience the event more as a playdate with a big person than an appointment to evaluate why she was less and less in command of her own language, and why, when I did arrange playdates, Lina wouldn't give her peers the time of the day.

"I believe Lina has a developmental language disorder," Dr. Brown informed me after the examination. "I want her to have an MRI and a hearing test and a speech evaluation. I know of a wonderful speech therapist at Rhode Island Hospital that I want to evaluate Lina."

Tears streamed as the reality of Lina's predicament set in yet a little further. It had all happened so quickly. It was almost impossible to believe that what the neurologist was describing had anything to do with my daughter.

"From the way you've described everything, I think you came here today blaming yourself for Lina's difficulties. I think this is way beyond circumstances. It's possible that her language difficulties are caused by the Epstein-Barr virus that she had in conjunction with the drooling episode at three-and-a-half. I measure language ability in four ways—naming, comprehension, repetition, and fluency. Apart from comprehension, which I don't have a clear sense of, Lina has difficulties in all areas."

Hearing Lina's fast footsteps and increasingly incoherent self-talking out in the waiting room (where I had left her under the supervision of Dr. Brown's secretary to avoid having to talk about Lina in front of her), I asked: "From what you've seen, how do you think I can best help Lina?"

He recommended that Lina receive intensive speech and language training for a couple of years. "Private school will most likely not accommodate her." He said, "Being able to utilize language is what makes us human. You want to get her a comprehensive IEP, an Individualized Educational Plan." Additionally, we discussed getting a developmental assessment and sensory integration treatment.

I had been trying to get her into the Meadowbrook Waldorf School, which was the system she knew best and had responded well to in the past.

"As long as she gets to work on her language," Dr. Brown stressed.

I was feeling very hopeful, and decided to pursue speech and language training in addition to sensory integration training. I started to look around for an occupational therapy clinic and began preparing for Lina's evaluation at a large Rhode Island hospital, by a speech therapist highly recommended by Dr. Brown. But when Lina and I walked into the waiting room, the receptionist apologized and told me that the speech pathologist unexpectedly had to attend a meeting but someone else would evaluate Lina. That someone else was one of the most disorganized professionals I have ever come across.

We entered his tiny, messy office, and the interview process began. While the speech pathologist chatted with me, Lina was soon climbing his desk and window, looking for something more interesting than the broken toys and torn puzzle pieces that were thrown in a pile on the floor in one corner of the room. At some point, the pathologist, let's call him Mr. K, attempted to entice Lina over to the corner with the broken toys to see if he could get a handle on her language skills. Lina stayed for a few minutes, unengaged, non-responsive, and soon Mr. K wrote that she operates on the level of a twenty-nine-month-old toddler. Fuming, I ended the interview process prematurely and left the office with Lina in my arms. Mr. K had recommended an MD, who specialized in helping children on the autism spectrum with language. When I later called to schedule an appointment with this doctor, his receptionist informed me that the doctor had stopped working with children with autism years ago. I sighed and kicked myself for leaving the civilization of New York City. Whether Lina had autism or didn't was still up for debate. No one had yet given her the diagnosis; in fact what we had most encountered so far were various professionals suggesting that Lina *didn't* have autism but something else—no one seemed to know exactly what—going on with her.

Lina's MRI was scheduled shortly after her speech evaluation. She first had to be sedated with a little prick in her arm
in order to facilitate injecting the IV that would put her to
sleep before sliding in under the MRI machine. The initial
sedation in the nurse's office was terrifying enough for Lina.
She calmed down for a while but the MRI team got preoccupied with something else and by the time they were ready
for her, she was beside herself and we ended up going home
without having completed the MRI. We came back a week
later. By this time Lina's terror of the little needle that would
calm her down enough to make possible the IV was ampli-
fied. It was heartbreaking. She fought with all the force her
little body could muster to ward off the team from injecting
the IV that would put her to sleep before the MRI. I held her
hand and kissed her and said, "Everything is going to be okay,
baby." She paused in her struggle for a moment, looked at me,
then at the nurse holding the needle and said, "Nej, det ar inte
okej." (No, it's not okay.)

I kissed and hugged her as she drifted off to sleep. As I saw
her little body being transported into the MRI machine,
I promised myself not ever to put my little girl through any
intrusive experiences like this unless absolutely necessary. It's
the worst part of being a parent—seeing in your child's eyes her
need for you to protect her, and her confusion about why you
won't. I felt so lonely and afraid, wanting desperately to pull her
out of that big, rumbling, plastic device and leave. I went to the
bathroom, had a good cry and came back, waiting for her to
come back to me. A week later, Dr. Brown called me and told
me that the MRI showed nothing. No "structural damage of the
brain." Now what?

More evaluations. We met with an occupational therapist at Therapediatrics in Kingston and had a period of occupational therapy there. I learned to brush her whole body in ways that seemed to help calm and focus her. In their sensory gym, Lina got to jump and slide, climb, swing and crawl, carry, and push. On the OT's recommendation, I ordered a heavy blanket for Lina to be wrapped up in at home and a heavy vest to wear on and off throughout the day.

The special educational team at Middletown public school, with their school psychologist performing a psychological evaluation, their educational specialist doing educational and cognitive testing, and their social worker writing up Lina's social history and tracking her development, led to a recommendation to their most intensive educational setting with only special kids. But other than the fact that all the kids had intense needs, the setting seemed to me not intense at all. Lina would have spent most of her time in the classroom, only occasionally being pulled out for one-on-one sessions for speech and occupational therapy. At this point, Lina would have been completely lost in a group setting, unable to sit still for more than a couple of minutes. Without ongoing one-on-one support, she would not focus on what was being said unless it was communicated directly to her. I rejected the setting after meeting with the prospective team, knowing that it wasn't nearly as vigorous a program as Lina needed.

I had noticed that the school psychologist, Sue Curley, had good rapport with Lina and was committed to the DIR (developmental, individual-difference, relationship-based) model developed by Dr. Stanley Greenspan. I was familiar with the work of this wonderful pediatrician, promoting a much more engaging and genuinely interactive approach to working with children with autism than the applied behavioral analysis (ABA) and other behavioral interventions that were normally prescribed to kids with these challenges. The DIR approach is often referred to as the Floortime model because a central aspect of this approach is to meet the child on his or her own developmental level and work on the foundations for development regardless of the child's age rather than focusing on outer behavior and symptoms. The most important and foundational learning, Dr. Greenspan stressed, takes place within the framework of meaningful, positive, and warm relationships. In contrast to DIR, ABA is focused mainly on the child's behavior. Instead of working within the context of the child's own motivation as in DIR and other relational models, ABA focuses on designing, implementing, and evaluating what environmental modifications can produce the most significant improvement in the child's behavior. ABA is built on a reward and punishment/consequence system where the child is rewarded if he or she answers and behaves correctly and suffers negative consequences if he answers and behaves incorrectly. "Incorrect" behavior may include stimming (self-stimulatory behavior, such as hand-flapping), very common in kids with autism, which is considered undesirable in spite of the fact that a child utilizes stimming to regulate his or her own often very disregulated feelings and sensations.

When I proposed, at the IEP meeting, that the school psychologist meet with Lina for floor time on a weekly basis, my suggestion was met with enthusiasm. Sue was fascinated by Lina's unusual presentation, and was clearly intrigued by the prospect of working with her. Later, though, as I followed up on this promising possibility, I was told that Dr. Curley had been transferred into another district. My request to have the public school reimburse me for working with Lina at home was rejected. Maybe I could have gotten somewhere with that had I insisted and fought with them and invested more time and energy on convincing the special education department that this was the most effective way of working with Lina. I decided instead on spending my energy and intelligence on how to best help Lina at this decisive time, and Tony and I agreed to pay for it ourselves.

To expand on my own understanding of what Lina was going through and evaluate the need for homeopathic medicine, Lina and I also met with an anthropologist and MD, Dr. Kelly Sutton. Dr. Sutton started Lina on a few different homeopathic remedies, including drops designed to restore balance in Lina's body and mind, which, ultimately, didn't seem to have much effect. Dr. Sutton's contribution to us was the words of understanding she communicated to me. It was a spiritual understanding and one that is so often missing in helping and treating children with autism: "I hear in your voice that you think it's too late. Don't think that. Maybe if you'd started Lina on all kinds of treatments sooner it would have broken her spirit. Maybe now she is ready. Lina is very brave to have chosen this path," she said. I looked at the tall, soft-spoken woman with her long hair in a thick braid down her back and felt the panic at the pit of my stomach subside. She looked at me sternly and said: "Don't regret anything. Trust what Lina is trying to do, that this is her destiny. She is lucky to have you fighting for her, doing everything you can to help her." I never forgot what she said. So often, for years after this meeting, I returned to this wise woman's words and found comfort. Trust what Lina is trying to do. Don't regret anything.

Lina and I also met with a well-known, very warm and intelligent female developmental pediatrician, Dr. Yatchmink, at the Children's Neurodevelopment Center at Rhode Island Hospital in Providence. After evaluating Lina, Dr. Yatchmink felt that Lina did not convincingly fit the picture of autism and recommended genetic testing. She told me that she thought Lina was much more related and in tune with her environment than the many kids on the autism spectrum that she had encountered. In the evaluation, Dr. Yatchmink wrote:

I did indicate to Lina's mother today that I am still uncertain about the etiology of Lina's autistic symptoms. I told her mother today that I am concerned about her significant history of regression and some of the atypical features of her behavioral profile and strongly recommended that Lina undergo a careful genetics evaluation to determine whether there might be a unifying etiology to explain her presentation.

Tony and I considered pursuing a genetics evaluation. But we didn't carry it through—it would have cost almost $10,000, only a quarter of which would be covered by insurance. We decided that our resources, at this time, were better spent on treating Lina, working with her, finding speech therapists and occupational therapists with innovative ideas, learning more about the various models available in treating and working with kids on the spectrum, and spending more time directly with Lina. We figured that putting Lina through genetic testing at this time, even if we did find something, was very unlikely to change the course of treatment.

I decided to take Lina to New York City to meet with two of the most sympathetic and astute neurodevelopment evaluators I have ever encountered. Together, Dr. Hahn-Burke, Psy.D., and Catherine Golding-Cremoux, MA, constitute a private New York City resource called PerDev (Perceptual Development). Lina, instantly sensing that this place was very different from some of the medical, clinical, and educational establishments she had walked in and out of in recent months, moved right into the evaluation playroom as if she instinctively knew that this was a place where she would be respected and taken seriously and that no one here would dream of forcing her to do anything. Uncharacteristically, she was fine with leaving me behind in the waiting room as long as she could occasionally skip back to check that I was still there.

On Lina's motor behavior, these evaluators wrote:

> *She was bold, but not reckless . . . demonstrated a range*
> *of different controlled gaits including running and some*
> *skipping . . . moved confidently on a variety of surfaces and*
> *grades . . . no vestibular uncertainty was noted. . . . She*
> *demonstrated control for a variety of fine motor skills.*

They noticed interesting inconsistencies in Lina's sensory responses:

> *She was extremely specific about where on her body she*
> *wanted to be held but she was only minimally responsive*
> *to gentle poking and rubbing of her back. . . . She did not*

respond to a loud siren of an ambulance going by on the street [part of the evaluation was outside]. She did, however, readily respond to the sound of the front entrance door of the office suite opening and closing . . . peeped outside . . . to see if her mother was still there.

On social and emotional behaviors, the evaluators wrote:

Although Lina did not participate in shared activities in an ongoing manner, she was aware of the consultants' presence and even turned to one of the more familiar consultants for physical contact.

Intensive speech and occupational therapy was recommended, as was dyadic, one-on-one psychotherapeutic work with the purpose of increasing regulatory capacities (holding it together emotionally, not falling apart), improving interpersonal relatedness, and expanding symbolic communication (helping Lina understand and work with more abstract language, in words and eventually in written language). A school or program with a small class size and high adult-to-student ratio was also recommended.

I left feeling that my daughter had been understood and appreciated. I had learned and re-learned things about her that would soon determine our choices for her future.

Alongside an ever-expanding evaluation process, I became possessed by the idea of creating a life for Lina. I wanted her to have more mutual friendships, illuminated teachers, and meaningful learning. The search for a good school became the way I tried to come to terms with what was happening with

Lina. I contacted the area's closest Waldorf school, an hour away from where we lived, and tried to the best of my ability to explain our somewhat unique situation. Teachers, board members, and a special-needs consultant were extremely receptive to us and we started the process of trying to determine whether Lina, and the rest of the Meadowbrook kids and teachers, would benefit or suffer from her increasingly hyperactive presence. In my mind, whether or not they welcomed Lina into their school became a prediction of whether she would be received and welcomed in the world. That was, of course, just my own little way of breaking down something about Lina's fate that was too difficult for me to metabolize at that time.

The first step was for Lina to visit an empty classroom with the head teacher at the school. To my surprise, Lina walked into the classroom, sat down by the table, and ate an entire apple without spitting out a single piece! Spitting out food, and picking it apart with her hands, was a relatively new behavior, but watching her now, eating her apple normally without doing anything to it apart from chewing and swallowing, made me very hopeful. As she ate her apple, she carefully observed the teacher and listened intently to her every word. Then she went over to the wooden play kitchen, feeding the teacher and her baffled mama pretend apples and plums and imagining that her friend Ellen was there with her. I was stunned, and even more convinced that a Waldorf school was what Lina needed. After a few days of panic, waiting for the school's decision, Mrs. Sky, the woman who would be Lina's head teacher, called and welcomed Lina for a three-day trial with the other kids. She wanted me—or, as she put it, "even better, someone else close, but not *so* close, to Lina"—to be there with her. I went to school with Lina the first day. The second and third day, Therese, the wonderful babysitter we'd had back in New York City, took the three-and-a-half-hour train ride from New York to Rhode Island to be by Lina's side as the Meadowbrook people determined her destiny. The three-day trial turned into a week trial, with the condition that we find a shadow, someone to work specifically with Lina in the classroom. The shadow would facilitate Lina's presence in the classroom and allow the other two teachers to go on with their teaching without too much disruption. It was an unusual situation. This particular Waldorf school was in the process of exploring the idea of integrating a small ratio of special needs children into their program. The school recommended Felicia as a candidate for the shadow position. She was already working at Meadowbrook and had a child with sensory processing issues. The week trial turned into a six-week trial. The six-week trial turned into a twelve-week trial, which brought us to the end of the spring semester.

Many things felt extremely important for all of us as we struggled through our Newport experience. And yet, for me, other than those first frightening months of Lina's most dramatic regression, nothing compared to the desperation I felt awaiting word on whether Lina would be invited to continue at Meadowbrook.

When we had invited Felicia to our house to be interviewed for the job of Lina's shadow, she stepped into the scene of Lina shredding paper, pouring milk and cereal on the floor, and climbing everything and everybody. None of this appeared to intimidate or discourage Felicia. Her hope and joyful enthusiasm was the sun breaking through dark clouds. I hired her as Lina's shadow on the spot.

Felicia turned out to be the only person, apart from Tony and myself, who was willing to care for both Lina and Elsa at the same time. Eventually, we started the tradition of me driving Lina and Elsa to Felicia's house one afternoon a week. They were to spend quality social time with Felicia and her six-year-old daughter Skyler. Soon even Felicia realized that this job needed a couple of extra pairs of hands and asked her husband to come home early from work those afternoons. Soon after that, Felicia's mother began to appear on those same afternoons, willing to offer her hands and heart to facilitate this challenging situation.

After Lina's initial three days in her new classroom, my dear friend Anki, who still had a few more months left in New York City before moving back to Sweden, brought Ellen, and Elsa's very close buddy Alfred, for a first visit to our new home. As always, Ellen loved everything her increasingly unusual friend Lina came up with. One day, Lauren came by for tea with her daughter Alicia, who was a few years older than Lina. Whether because of Lina's difficulties or the fact that Alicia was a little older, their connection was solely based on the fact that their parents were good friends. I had never really seen the two playing together. And now, Lina walked up to Alicia, who was standing in the middle of the living room, looked straight at her and said, "This is Alicia. Do I know her? No!"

For a couple of moments everyone stopped what they were doing, as if to determine how to react to this statement. Then Ellen, the true friend that she is, broke the ice and burst out laughing. She found the comment hilarious. Anki and I looked at each other and then joined Ellen, laughing until tears were rolling down our cheeks. I felt so grateful for this little girl's ability to appreciate life just as it presented itself to us, helping us all to find joy in this new and unusual situation. Lina was changing in front of our eyes. Most of the time, I went to bed each night and woke up every morning with the same excruciating sense of terror. I lived with a sense of being encapsulated in a nightmare that for some incomprehensible reason didn't end, but just escalated. But with little Ellen there, and the warm feeling of us all being together again, watching Lina sitting opposite her best friend in the soft afternoon sun by the big wooden table cutting up clay in little tiny pieces, life seemed possible again. One of the last nights before Anki, Ellen, and Alfred were to head back to New York City, Lina and Elsa and I were lying in our bedroom before going to sleep. Elsa turned to me and said, "I love you. *Jag alskar dig och jag alskar* Lina."

"*Jag alskar Elsa* (I love Elsa)," Lina responded softly.

"*Mamma, hon sa det!* (Mama, she said it!") Elsa almost shouted out in excitement.

Had Elsa not noticed and reacted so strongly to those magical words, I would not have believed what I had just heard. I did not know that this would be my daughter's last verbal expression of love for a very long time. Thankfully, I had no way of predicting that this was more of a loving goodbye to her little sister before a long, difficult journey into herself, than the hopeful comeback we then anticipated. But I often feel grateful that Lina was able to tell Elsa this. And I have reminded Elsa innumerable times of that moment, so as to help her not to forget that even when Lina often seems far away from us, she loves her little sister very much. And Elsa, craving her big sister's love, hung onto every word.

That same evening, faithful to an old tradition, Anki and I were sitting downstairs after all of our children finally had fallen asleep, sipping tea and eating Trader Joe's milk chocolate with almonds. We celebrated the love Lina had managed to express to her sister. Unable to look at the situation in any other way, I had decided that we were going to get Lina back. We weren't going to let sensory processing disorder, expressive language disorder, autism, or anything else steal her away from us. There would be a day when all of our children would play together like they had in the past. Being expressive and creative, arguing and making up, writing letters to each other, asking each other questions and responding to them—all of it would one day become a reality again. At that time, I had no other way of conceptualizing what was happening to Lina. I couldn't let go of hope. I didn't think there was any other way of relating to Lina's challenges. How can you accept the unacceptable? Now, I know that it all starts there. Living each day with full acceptance of what is, while at the same time doing the very best with every moment that comes your way.

It was bittersweet to watch Lina and Ellen together, to watch Ellen's ongoing attempts to engage and interact with her friend. Lina's inexplicable loss of peace, language, eye contact, and ability to play must have been painful for Ellen. Though Lina seemed oblivious and unable, most of the time, to respond, Ellen accepted and still wholeheartedly admired her friend, who reminded her of the bold, unconventional, and good-hearted Swedish fairytale figure Pippi Longstocking. Dropping our friends off at the train station the next day, located an hour away from our house, I swallowed hard to fight back the big lump in my throat that threatened to explode into a thousand uncontrollable tears. Our family needed this family around. What was I doing, trying to build a community up on a New England island where everyone except us seemed to be related and the only family that we knew up here didn't want my daughter in their house? It began to seem as if I was making a lot of bad choices. Relating to the challenging situation by questioning my choices wasn't very productive. But to trust myself during this time seemed so difficult. On the inside, as I was trying to get used to the fact that Lina was no longer the Lina I had known, everything felt so out of control. Crossing the bridges on our way back home from the train station, I wondered how we would make it through the afternoon before bedtime. Maybe if we start with snack, I thought to myself, then we'll swing, then we'll listen to music and dance, and then, when everything begins to fall apart and Lina gets restless and starts pouring shampoo, eating toothpaste, snatching foods, and eating crayons, I'll put the girls in the car and go for a ride, while singing along to the girls' favorite CDs.

Every day was the same. I needed to make detailed plans in order to get us through. Lina was spending three mornings a week in school. The afternoons following such mornings were pure hell. Maybe Lina, not capable of processing the challenges of a group and school setting, held it together the best she could before coming home. She had meltdowns in school as well, but more often, she would let it out in the car on the way home. She would scream so loud that Elsa would cover her ears with her little chubby hands and cry. Lina would scream, hit me and sometimes Elsa in the face, do her usual pouring and ripping with escalated intensity, run out in the yard, pee and poop in the frozen flower beds, laugh in a loud, hollow manner that made me picture her alone in a cold, echoing stone cave, losing her mind and experiencing her life so devoid of feelings and human contact that hollow laughter was the only thing left. As I was chasing after Lina, Elsa would panic, cry, and beg me to stay inside.

"I'm sorry, Elsa, I'll be back," I would tell her as I ran out the door. "We'll figure something out," was my standard phrase to her. This period in our life was so overwhelming that it seemed impossible to remember anything before or hope for anything after. There were dark days and pitch-dark days. One day, as we were driving home after one of Lina's school days, approaching the first bridge taking us back to the island, Lina's screaming seemed louder and more detached than ever. Suddenly, in the middle of a busy highway, I witnessed in the rear-view mirror how she managed to Houdini her way out of her car seat and jump up to the seat next to me, trying to open the glove compartment to see if there were any hidden goodies inside. I pulled over to the shoulder of the road, emergency blinkers on, feeling my heart pumping and adrenaline shooting through my body.

"LINA, WHAT THE HELL ARE YOU DOING? STAY IN YOUR GODDAMN SEAT!" I screamed at her. Not knowing what to do with the panicky feelings raging through my body, I got out, slammed the door, and continued screaming. "THIS IS TOO CRAZY! GOD, HELP US, I CAN'T DO THIS, WHAT THE HELL DO YOU EXPECT FROM ME?" I walked toward the back of the car, crying and asking the higher powers to help me. As I was standing there, with a scared Elsa inside the car and with Lina oblivious as to why I suddenly started to yell at her, I wondered why God seemed to take such special care in demonstrating to me how abandoned I was by everything and everybody. I tried reasoning. "Why do you need to keep showing me how exposed I am? I've always known it. What did I do to *you*?" Another eternal five minutes went by before I was able to open the car door, put Lina back in her seat, and drive home.

"Mama, why did you leave? Why did you get angry and cry?" Elsa wanted to know. Lina didn't say anything; she just stared out the window, laughing to herself.

"It's so dangerous to move around in the car when we're driving. I'm sorry that I screamed at you, Lina. I was so afraid when you got out of the car seat." I turned to Elsa, trying to explain what had just happened.

"See, sometimes when people get really afraid, they seem angry. I wasn't really angry at Lina, just very afraid when she got out of her seat. We always have to stay in our seats. We'll have to come up with something." The next day, I went to Walmart to buy a car seat made for a younger child, knowing that we wouldn't be able to drive anywhere if Lina wasn't securely fastened in her seat.

With increasing frequency, Lina started to try to leave the house. Tony came by my house early each Friday morning to pick up the girls so that I could catch the first train to New York City and see my clients. During this time, I came back before, or during, Lina and Elsa's bedtime preparations. I would drive by Tony's house and pick them up in their pajamas, already fed and bathed. Then Saturday morning, Elsa would go over to Tony's house for some peaceful one-on-one time with him, and Lina and I would hang out, just the two of us. Tony's house had a door that opened right onto a busy street. He put a big couch on the inside in front of the door and used his balcony door to get in and out of the house. My street was calmer. Both Tony and I, and, unfortunately and unfairly, Elsa, became experts in knowing exactly where Lina was at any given time, day and night.

But along with our growing collective hypervigilance, Lina developed a strange sixth sense of when, exactly, an opportunity for escape became available. One day, Elsa and I were in the kitchen, finishing up lunch. Lina had gone to the bathroom. Suddenly, I realized how quiet everything was. I no longer heard the toilet seat squeaking and her mumbling to herself. I rushed from the table, ran over to the tiny bathroom next to the living room; no Lina.

"LINA!" I immediately shouted, feeling the panic spreading through my stomach like wildfire. I ran upstairs. No Lina. The familiarity of the situation felt like a mountain on my chest. Four steps at a time down the stairs, back to Elsa in the kitchen. "Elsa, stay here and finish your apple, I'm just going to run outside to look for Lina. Okay?"

"Okay, Mama."

She was not in the yard. The street was empty. Randomly and without much time to think, I picked the most likely direction. The next hundred yards might have been record-breaking. I was down at the next street in less than ten seconds and turned right, on instinct. Half a block down the next street, with much more traffic and danger for Lina, I saw a police car pulled up and a woman holding my daughter's hand talking to the policeman. I was there with my arms around Lina in less than a heartbeat. Sweat dripped down my forehead and I was gasping for air. I just held my little girl as tears again flooded my cheeks. The sympathetic policeman followed us home, recorded the incident, and promised to stay sensitive to the possibility that he may run into Lina again. There was no judgment, no words of advice, and I felt like I'd just won the lottery. My daughter back, an understanding, compassionate policeman, and a neighbor who'd handed my daughter over to me with nothing but a relieved smile. This was good.

Another positive consequence of living in Newport was that in the midst of all the difficulties, Lina, Elsa, and I became a team. In the absence of the community we'd come there to build, we might as well have lived alone on that small, desolated island next to Newport Bridge. Together, we coordinated what to eat, when to swing, when to take a car ride to some new and interesting playground or go to the beach (which eventually didn't work so well, since Lina had a habit of leaping out of the car as soon as we got to the beach and sprinting straight out into the water, winter, spring, summer, and fall). On Valentine's Day, we celebrated with heart-shaped gingersnap cookies, pancakes, and popcorn. We listened to lots of love songs and Lina and I even had a little moment, just her and me, on a little playground next to a big wheat field as Elsa fell asleep in the car. Our sweet celebration of love reminded me that now I could create our life together in whatever way I believed was necessary and good. I no longer had to wait or negotiate or argue or engage someone else. Our life would become whatever we turned it into. I felt a sense of freedom. It motivated me to take every situation, even trivial ones, in Elsa's and Lina's and my life very seriously. Every meal that could be finished without food being thrown or cups shattered became a reason to celebrate. Every opportunity to help Lina engage with her little sister—who was desperate to have her back to answer her questions, go down the slide with her, dance to "Africa" together with her on the floor rather than in my arms, splash water with her in the bathtub—mattered more than ever.

I experienced this period as a matter of losing Lina or getting her back. Time was utterly important. It had to happen now.

Our life was so intense that most of the time I had no opportunity to worry about how isolated we had become. Sometimes, circumstances threw me a reminder. Lina and Elsa and I were hanging out at a nearby playground. As often during the weekdays in the cold season, we were the only ones there. Except for a middle-aged man who sat on a park bench nearby, observing us. At some point, I became aware of his interest. In spite of a strange feeling in my stomach, I nodded and tried a friendly smile in his direction. He smiled back, but his smile seemed cold. I turned to my girls and explained that we would need to get back home to make dinner in about five minutes. The man kept watching as we packed up our things and climbed into the car. Then he stood up and walked fast over to his car. I started mine. He started his. I waited. He waited. I turned out of the driveway onto the road. The man followed. I waited. He waited. I drove to my house, scolding myself for overreacting. I drove into our driveway, noticing in the back mirror that the man was still with us. He hesitated, slowed down, and then sped up again. I sat there in the driver's seat wondering about my own judgment. What am I thinking, a single mother of two girls escorting this man to our house? I called my friend Michael and asked him to keep his cell phone handy. "It's nothing," I reassured him, "but I just want to know that I can reach you."

"Do you want me to come over?"

"No, and whatever you do, don't tell Tony. Just keep your cell phone on." I didn't want Tony to worry. In New York City, four hours away, there wasn't much he could do. And I never saw the man again.

At times, we dealt with the sense of isolation and loss in Rhode Island by visiting our friends in New York City. It was intense to travel with Lina on the train, but trying to maintain the connection with what was familiar and safe was more important than whether or not we annoyed a few co-passengers on the MTI train. Many people had trouble with Lina's lack of social consciousness. With lightning speed, she would run up to people in the aisle, and before I had the chance even to notice that she had left her seat, she would have grabbed somebody's cookie or French fry or piece of candy. With me having recently implemented a gluten-free, dairy- (casein) free and sugar-free diet, short of knocking her down on the floor, I would shout, whistle, jump, dive, and knock other people over to prevent her from putting one of those foods in her mouth. She was fast and I had to be faster. My passion for beach volleyball with diving and defense as my specialty came in handy.

Gluten in particular stays in the system long after it's ingested, and the effect in children with autism, who frequently have trouble breaking down the protein found in gluten, is often devastating, including more hyperactivity, screaming, stomach aches, and compromised language and eye contact. The same is often true for casein, a protein found in dairy. The effect that sugar had on Lina was the most immediate. Ingesting sugary foods, including brown sugar, agave, honey, and maple syrup, gave Lina a five-minute high followed by hours of misery. Lina had always liked sweet foods, but since she began to lose her developmental abilities at three and a half, she had craved sugar with a vengeance. And she always responded to it with tears, screams, and increasingly out-of-control and erratic behavior. Sugar, more than anything else, is not Lina's friend. So, I didn't, and still don't, have many qualms about knocking a few people over or startling some others in my quest to keep Lina off the foods that hurt her.

For as long as Anki and her family were still living in New York City, we would periodically visit them at their house on the Upper West Side. We would celebrate our reunions with our traditional pasta (now made of brown rice) with meat sauce and Anki and I would have red wine and make toasts for our beautiful children and our solid friendship. Anders, her husband, would be off traveling to some far-away country for his work at UNICEF, and Anki and I, faithful to our traditions, would finish our days with tea and chocolate and talking and laughing for many hours after our four children had all fallen asleep. We would talk about Lina's recovery and our children's deep friendship with each other. We would compare notes on our marital experiences and laugh about my intense personality and Anki's tendency to constantly be the mediator and facilitator for everyone around her. These evenings helped me to reconnect with a time when I wasn't just a terrified mother of a child with increasing special needs.

Despite my intention to make one such visit the same as it always was, things during our children's spring break turned out very differently. As soon as Lina and Elsa and I put down our bags inside our friends' apartment, I took one look at Anki and realized something wasn't right.

"You look terrible," I told my friend.

"I think I'm okay, just a little tired."

"What's the matter with you? Your face is green! Go lie down, for God's sake!" I demanded. Reluctantly, Anki dragged her feet into the bedroom. She had already prepared dinner so it was ready for us to sit down and eat. Apart from having to get up to chase Anki into the bedroom where she belonged, dinner, miraculously, was doable. And bath time, with all four kids overcrowding the tub, was almost like the old days.

The next afternoon, it was my and Lina's turn to feel weak and helpless. Poor Anki, far from recovered, appeared with her pale face in our bedroom in the middle of the night before I made it to the bathroom for my first upwardly mobile "deposit." Without the will power to chase her away this time, I let her be there, next to me, with extra towels and sheets and her extra hands, ready and wholehearted as always. Lina threw up in the bed before any of us had the chance to blink and the night became a race between the bathroom and the bedroom, sometimes for me, sometimes for Lina, sometimes for the two of us.

Amazingly, Elsa never got sick and in a few days the three of us, Lina and I a couple of pounds lighter, were ready to hop on the train back to Rhode Island. This time, Tony came with us on the train since he had been working in the city and was on his way back for the weekend. While things were still tense between Tony and me, the intensity of trying to figure out and relate to what was happening to our oldest daughter forced us to cooperate in spite of our decision to separate from each other. The reality of us being apart began to sink in. At the same time, in the context of Lina's development and difficulties, the anger and pain between Tony and me, our life-changing decision to go separate ways after our fifteen years together, quickly was pushed into a peripheral corner of our lives. We didn't have time to worry too much about who was right and who was wrong. We barely had time to brush our teeth, much less to figure out the psycho-dynamics of our failed marriage. In retrospect, I think that was one of the many gifts our unusual and intense daughter gave to us. A lot of things can go wrong when a hyperactive four-and-a-half-year-old is left unsupervised for a few minutes. Cereal can be dumped all around the kitchen, crayons can be eaten, little sister can be bitten, toothpaste eaten, body lotion spread all over the bed, the dining table peed on, and, worst of all, the child can find a way to get out of the house during those five minutes and disappear! There was no time to dwell on the past.

Due to the sheer pressure and unpredictability of the situation, anxiety and panic became almost everyday states. I had to develop ways to live with chaos and started to do daily yoga, tiptoeing out the bedroom door before sunrise, praying that the girls would stay asleep. If that failed, I would find my yoga mat in the evening after my girls went to sleep. I also started to pray. Not to the punitive, persecutory, humiliating God I had grown up with, but to God in everyone, to God that's in the water splashing up on the cliffs by the beach where I ran to every chance I got, God that's in the wind that makes gentle whispering melodies as it blows through the leaves, God that's in the sun that warms up our cold souls after long winters. I began to pray to the God that is love between people—connecting me and my little four-and-a-half-year-old beautiful troublemaker, consoling the pain between me and Tony, healing my relationship with my dying mother, preserving and strengthening the bond between Elsa and Lina and between me and my dear friends. Love, God, yoga, praying, crying and laughing every chance I got, as well as the hours and hours on the quiet winter beaches of Newport and Middletown, helped me through this strenuous time with more sanity than what I had started with.

After a lot of ambivalence, I decided that it was important for me to keep on working with the people to whom I had committed and to continue my part-time practice in New York. Up until now I had been going back and forth every Friday. Now I started to stay over in New York City on Friday nights in order to see a few more clients in the city on Saturday mornings. Dropping the girls off at Tony's house that first early Friday morning of my new arrangement, I felt so torn apart. I simply couldn't fight off the tears as I kissed Lina goodbye to be away from her overnight for the first time ever. It seemed like the wrong time in her life to leave her behind. It was a little easier with Elsa since I knew she wasn't as impacted by the separation. The train rides to the city became daytime opportunities to reach doctors and schedule evaluations, talk to teachers and find babysitters, make notes about Lina and think things through. I found a Defeat Autism Now (DAN) doctor on one of those train rides.

CHAPTER FOUR

Diet and Playroom

His name is Darren Lynch. Like his DAN colleagues all around the country, he devotes his innovative practice to biomedical diagnosis and treatment, prescriptions of supplements, diet, anti-yeast treatment, antiviral treatments, B12 injections, chelating testing and treatment, nicotine patches, and anything else under the sun that's worth trying to calm down, refocus, perk up, and improve eye contact, language, and gastrointestinal health of so many young patients on the spectrum. We did not yet have a diagnosis for Lina, but the possibility that she might have autism was difficult to ignore.

We started the complicated process of collecting and shipping Lina's blood, urine, and stool to all kinds of different laboratories all around the United States. Collecting Lina's blood and poop was a nerve-wracking, long, drawn-out affair. One stool test needed to be collected on three different occasions, stored, and then shipped before its expiration date. I remember driving off with record-breaking speed into the night trying to get to a DHL office off the island, halfway to Providence, since failing to get there before the pickup time would force us to collect new, fresher samples for another three days. I simply couldn't face intruding on Lina anymore and didn't care if I lost my driver's license in the process. All that mattered was that I got this sacred package to the laboratory. I pleaded with the DHL staff to keep their doors open for me for another five minutes while internally I resolved to move back to New York City where there would be UPS, DHL, and FedEx offices around most corners, regardless of where we lived.

Nothing dramatic came out of any of the tests, but that didn't discourage Dr. Lynch from starting Lina on supplements such as the probiotic *Saccharomyces boulardi*, taurine (a protein that kids with autism often don't have enough of and that can have a calming effect), zinc, magnesium, dimethylglycine (DMG), folinic acid, B12 injections (stimulating eye contact, language, and general learning and relatedness), twice yearly very high dose of vitamin A to see if we could get rid of the viral issues that I suspected were in Lina's system, theanine (protein contributing to well-being), anti-yeast powder, and many other biomedical remedies. We also tried B6 vitamins, which we hoped would help Lina with producing neurotransmitters. Even though we gave Lina B6 in combination with magnesium to help prevent the increasing hyperactivity and biting often associated with B6, the magnesium didn't sufficiently slow Lina down. So we discontinued the B6 after Lina's biting habits worsened and I, fighting to hold back tears from increasingly painful, much deeper bite marks and an injured heart, called Dr. Lynch's nurse for advice. Without even consulting the doctor, she immediately suggested that I stop giving Lina the B6 supplement. I did. Biting subsided.

Life became focused on how to make a gluten-, casein-, and sugar-free diet appealing and tasty while at the same time concealing the bitter taste of multiple supplements by adding them to pancakes or baking them into muffins and scones and strange-tasting cookies. Mealtimes inevitably became more stressful. Up to this point I had always operated with the idea that becoming over-invested in your child's eating is not a good idea. It invites power struggles. Being faithful to this idea and offering good, healthy foods without elements of reward or punishment for eating or not eating them had always worked well. Both Lina and Elsa have learned to love the taste of broccoli, whole-grain bread, rice and beans, and sprouts and cabbage without much prompting from me and Tony. Now, suddenly, I stunned Lina by demanding that she eat the pancake with the supplement mix on top before the next pancake. Until Dr. Lynch had warned me about the yeast-producing components of all kinds of sweeteners, including agave nectar, honey, and authentic maple syrup, I poured those sweet enticers over everything I wanted Lina to eat. The bitter taste of her anti-yeast powder was nearly impossible to conceal. The raspberry-tasting liquid folinic acid with extra B12 in it was a big help until they stopped manufacturing it due to the fact that it was not efficiently absorbed in a liquid form.

I believe that all those measures, in combination, were helpful to Lina. Things gradually got noticeably better. Lina did okay during her mornings at the Waldorf school and, after a meeting with teachers, the school counselor, and the director of the school board, the school welcomed Lina to continue in the small class, called "middle school" in Waldorf language, for another trial year. We were very happy about that possibility. Yet, during that summer, I thought a lot about the intensity of Lina's services. She saw her OT once weekly and her speech therapist three times a week. It wasn't enough. She was almost five and learning centers in her brain were still flexible enough to allow radical improvements. I wanted more for her. So I decided to take her out of the Waldorf school and work with her myself, at home.

The frustrating and disappointing process of trying to attain adequate support from the public school system on the island strengthened my resolve in taking full responsibility for Lina's recovery myself. I knew Tony would support me once he realized the benefits. I researched the Web for more innovative, relational approaches to autism than the existing ABA (applied behavioral analysis) that most pediatricians, teachers, and social workers swore by.

A few months earlier, Tony had come across an article about the Son-Rise Program of the Austism Treatment Center of America. It was founded by Barry and Samahria Kaufman, who reached and found a cure for their own son with severe symptoms of autism through their hard, intense, and love-driven work. Their son Raun, who is now a central part of the Son-Rise Program, teaching and giving lectures all around the globe on how to help kids with autism, was in much worse shape than Lina. At the age of one,

Raun withdrew from human contact. By the age of four, after years of his parents' intensive, one-on-one work with him, guided by unconditional love and acceptance, Raun's symptoms disappeared. The idea behind The Son-Rise Program is to encourage and motivate parents and volunteers to spend intensive, enthusiastic, and present time with the child in a playroom free from the distractions of life around them. The program is part of the Option Institute in Sheffield, Massachusetts, focusing on counseling and instructing families on how to create their own, home-based programs for their own special children.

As I read about this philosophy, I felt a sense of relief. This approach to autism had so much more to do with building relationships with children who have difficulties in this area than rewarding and punishing desired or undesired behaviors. Sure, every child is different. But I didn't want Lina just to behave age-appropriately. It would be nice if she sometimes didn't automatically do the opposite of what we were asking her. And I didn't enjoy the screaming and the biting and the running after her down the street. I dreaded spending three hours at bedtimes, with her running around the small bedroom laughing and screaming before going to bed. But if I had to choose between having a relationship with her or having her be accommodating but not genuinely connected and engaged, I would always choose the relationship. The most painful part of autism, for me, is to lose the one you love so much while she is just in front of you.

Inspired by the Son-Rise model, I turned our bedroom upstairs into a playroom, free from the distractions of the rest of the house. The tiny upstairs guest room became Lina's, Elsa's, and my new bedroom. All the pictures and drawings, little lamps, and bright-colored curtains that I had put up in our former bedroom to make the space cozy and homelike came down. I wanted to help my overstimulated, hyperactive little girl to calm down. I wanted to create enough peace and simplicity in there to enable us to find each other again. And I wanted to give Lina a good time. So often, Lina's life became a constant confrontation with everybody else's attempt to stop her from whatever it was she was doing. Everyone around her always said, "NO." Almost everything she wanted to do was out of her reach and met with reservation and limit-setting. And the irony was that in her current state of development, Lina wasn't socially invested enough to respond to our protests. So this playroom, in order to become a source of connection and healing, had to represent something welcoming and affirmative for her. And I was dying to be with her in a space where I would be in a position to go along with her initiatives rather than constantly having to prevent her from doing what she wanted to do.

I furnished the playroom with only a children's table and two chairs and bought a small trampoline, a bouncing ball, and a thick mat that would cushion our knees when we were hanging out on the floor together. Then I brought in the CD player and all of Lina's favorite music, clay and a bunch of tools for the clay, some of Lina's favorite books, and a few puppets. Whenever possible, Lina and I started to spend time together up in the playroom. We always brought snacks that Lina and I picked out together beforehand. And, miraculously, Lina, who is the most freedom-hungry little child I have ever met and who despised being confined to any area designed by someone else, accepted our time in there with very little protest. As children so often do, she quickly recognized the opportunities of this room and time together. Music, bouncing on the ball, jumping on the trampoline, cutting clay, snacking, popping bubble wrap, and roughhousing and tickling games on the mat became the most popular playroom activities. Already, on our third playroom session, Lina ran ahead of me up the stairs and into the playroom as soon as I told her we were going. We cut peaches and nectarines together and suddenly Lina jumped up from the table and around the room, shouting some made-up words, louder and louder. I jumped up from my seat and started jumping and shouting along with her. Lina stopped in the middle of one of her jumps, looked straight into my eyes, and smiled. It was a turning point. The panic at the pit of my stomach slowly subsided. Lina's smile became more frequent and socially meaningful and the biting, little by little, began to disappear.

Whenever Lina got disregulated, showing more hyperactive, erratic, and impulsive behavior, she benefited from tight embraces and some bouncing on the large blow-up ball or me moving around with her in my arms for a few minutes. She loved piggyback rides and, if facing me as I held her, to turn her head away from me and hide it between my shoulders and chin. As soon as she relaxed, she would lift her head up and gaze into my eyes with the most meaningful, warm smile. When she was on my back, I'd bring her in front of the mirror and we'd look into each other's eyes through the mirror. This indirect eye contact, via the mirror, helped Lina to remain engaged and looking at me for longer and longer periods. This in itself, after the past difficult months of less and less direct eye contact, felt to me as if I was getting my daughter back. From here, looking into each other's eyes, feeling connected and close, everything started.

We spent a lot of time dancing and singing to the music in front of the mirror, just being together and getting closer again. During this period, Lina's favorite songs were "I can sing, I can sing, I can do almost anything!" and a song about a melancholic horse in need of an attitude transformation. The horse didn't think he could do things but was encouraged to "try, just try." Maybe Lina was inspired by the messages of these songs? She was suddenly in a position where I asked her for so much more. I wanted to give her ongoing chances to find her way back to her own words. And I wanted her to experience the very real and immediate rewards of communication. And I hoped to help her understand how important she was to me. I wanted her to know that when we were in the playroom together, nothing else mattered. Everything outside had to wait. No cell phones were on, nobody disturbed us when we were together in the playroom. All that existed was the two of us, finding new and old ways to connect, communicate, and have fun. Lina's ability to pretend and her capacity for symbolic play, such as making food out of clay, resurfaced.

I kept a journal of every session, keeping them as brief and descriptive as I could. August 8, 2008, was typical of the sessions that first month in the playroom:

> *9 a.m. to 10:30 a.m. Playing with new Play-Doh, Lina labels the white Play-Doh and eventually pink and brown Play-Doh. Keeps asking for black Play-Doh. Describes to me how she is cutting the Play-Doh "in half," and "two pieces," and "three pieces." Occasionally gives me a piece. Pretends the Play-Doh is pasta and cuts "pieces of bacon" and gives me a piece. Not interested in dress up today. Bites me, I gently push her away. Listens to music and chooses the "Yes, I can" song over the others. Has fun with raisins and runs around with them. I pretend to be a monkey, chasing her and begging for raisins and she laughs and tries to get away. Likes to be rolled up in a blanket. Laughs, rolled up on the*

*floor and looks at me, then smiles softly. More music, likes
to be held close. Laughs when I jump up and down with
her, rolls down from being held to hanging upside down, me
holding onto her legs. Wants to do this several times.*

In order to spend this time with Lina, I needed to make plans
for Elsa. Janet, a beautiful young mother of four-year-old Oliver
and two-year-old Morgan, responded to an ad for babysitting
that Tony and I had put out on Craigslist. Her husband was a
full-time trumpet player in the U.S. Navy band and Janet was
home taking care of her boys. I instantly liked Janet's warm, subtle,
and gentle presence and together we agreed that Elsa, who at
two and a half was in desperate need of playmates, would spend
three mornings a week with Janet and her boys while I worked
with Lina in the playroom. The other two mornings, Elsa spent
with Mrs. Monegan, a Waldorf teacher receiving young children
in her home, where homemade bread, a large vegetable garden,
wooden toys, and trees all around the property provided Elsa
with the retreat she needed from everyday challenges at home.
At Mrs. Monegan's, Elsa found Lily, her very first best girlfriend.

And Lina, after we dropped Elsa off, found rotten apples and
peaches on the ground in the extended garden next to where
parents parked their cars. Her fascination with only the rotten
fruit, and her wish to squeeze it and smush it up as much as she
could and then smear it all over her clothes, initially bothered me.
Why wouldn't she want the good fruit? Why did everything have
to be the opposite of what one would generally expect? But then
I had to ask myself, "Do I really want to get to know my girl? Am
I really willing to be in her world or is it more important for me
to make her be in ours?" The answer, to me, was obvious and often
very challenging. Soon, I was crawling around on the ground

with her, trying to find the most rotten peaches, squeezing and poking them just like she did. It became what we did right after dropping off Elsa. Lina did appreciate my efforts. Her flickering glances over in my direction became more extended. Her smiles more frequent. Her little songs more audible. It was so wonderful to experience this quiet connection and understanding between us while at the same time knowing that Elsa was playing with her new friends, eating homemade bread, gathering vegetables, and taking long nature walks in a home that was characterized by love and genuine awareness of what children truly need.

Very quickly, the increasing relatedness became apparent not just in the playroom but also when Lina and Elsa and I were together. I wanted to add more hours in the playroom but also wanted to have much-needed one-on-one time with Elsa, who had to accommodate way too much to the difficulties of our situation. Tony put another ad on Craigslist for babysitters willing to work with special-needs children and one day Valerie walked in our door. She had an almost visible emotional sturdiness and a fearless attitude in relating to Lina, who was unusually hyped up by the number of visitors dropping by our house that afternoon, and who literally and figuratively climbed the walls, windows, and staircase as Valerie calmly watched her. I hired Valerie on the spot and she accepted with a smile as if that was exactly what she had expected and prepared for. I also asked Janet if she would be willing to do some playroom hours with Lina at times when her husband was home to take care of her boys. Janet, with her humble, loving, and soft joyfulness, was the first person other than myself to connect with Lina in the playroom. Lina accepted her presence instantly. Together, they looked at pictures in the picture albums, played with clay, and danced to the music.

I started an official playroom book where everyone working with Lina could observe and record their own and others' work. The book was introduced with:

Lina, my Love,
My wonderful, mysterious, sensitive, lovely, and loving little
girl. I have faith that everyone writing in this book, everyone
who has the awesome opportunity to get to know you, to
really get you, will fall in love.
Your very happy mother.

I suspect every mother feels something similar to this. But to be together with Lina, without any other concerns than to have a good time with her and be in the present moment, seemed to have a transformative effect not just on Lina and me, but on everyone who had the opportunity to be with her there. I advertised at a nearby university to see if I could find students who would be interested in hearing more about how to do relational playroom work with a child on the spectrum and got a big response. Eventually, innovative, charming, and charismatic Jackie started to come to our house a couple of times a week to be with Lina in the playroom. Soft-spoken, loyal, and thoughtful Maryanne was another student from the university who started to come and work with Lina a couple of hours a week. Then Susan, a native Rhode Islander with a gleam in her eye and a big heart, started to divide her time between playing with Lina in the playroom and taking Elsa for playdates with her eight-year-old daughter. Lina still talks about "riding in Susan's car." Susan had a big SUV with a giant, loud, and enthusiastic dog in the backseat. Innumerable times, in summer, fall, and winter, Susan took Lina to the beach and came back an hour later with a drenched Lina and, yes, since she had to chase after my very speedy daughter to get her out of the water, a very wet Susan as well.

In the midst of this dramatic time, I took the girls to Sweden to spend time with my mother. Our good friend Michael agreed to come with me. This was the first time Michael had met my family and they all loved him. Lina and Elsa, too, loved having him around and it reminded me of how easy it can be to have another adult person there with you at all times. Somehow, contrary to expectation, Lina did beautifully during these two weeks that for me involved sadness about my mother's rapidly progressing cancer. Walking in through the door of my parents' house and catching the first glimpse of my mother standing there, so frail and tired, so different from her usual energetic, fast-paced, powerful physical presence, now leaning up against the wall for support, made it all real. I was glad to be there. And I decided instantly to let go of every thought of regret for everything that had and hadn't happened between us, and focus on learning as much as I could about my mother and spending as much time with her as possible for these two weeks that we did have together.

We quickly settled into a routine of pancake breakfasts, swimming in a nearby lake, blueberry picking in the forest a mile from my parents' house, late lunches, more excursions, and dinners around ten or eleven at night. Somehow Lina listened better than I had seen in many months and also started to form "I" sentences like "I really like raspberries." My mother's anxiety about having plants, books, and albums ripped to pieces by Lina did heighten my little five-year-old's incentive to figure out what else she could do to make her grandmother lose her cool. It was amazing to see how dramatically Lina's language improved. I am still not sure why.

Could it have been the fact that we were all gathered in a house together with all the relatives and people around her that vitalized her language? Maybe all the swimming and berry picking? Whatever it was, it didn't last after our return to Newport, though we continued to go to the beach as often as we could.

Lina has always loved water. Whenever I had one-on-one time with Lina and we were maxed out in the playroom, I drove us to the beach. There are several beaches on Aquidneck Island. First beach and Second beach were the closest to our house. Second beach was longer and less populated. The sand on Second beach was soft and deep, with sand dunes surrounding the beach and making it a protected, serene place that instantly calmed Lina down. On one side of the beach were rocks that made the ideal climbing gym for Lina. She and I climbed up and down those rocks every chance we got. Hand in hand, we jumped from rock to rock, learning to keep our balance and take each other's movements into account. Together, we would stand at the highest point of the rocks, looking out onto the water, watching the birds soar, playing in the wind near the surface, or looking at the windsurfers, ceaselessly trying to follow the wind and stay just above or below the breaking point of the waves, falling, climbing up again, getting their rides, losing them, coming up on the beach, warming up in their pickup trucks, going back into the water, starting all over.

Most days, Lina and I would just wander up and down the beach, looking for seaweed, the green and the red kind with air-filled bubbles that pop like little balloons when you squeeze them or, as Lina often preferred, bite down on them. And then suddenly, in a moment of spontaneous happiness and inspiration, winter and summer alike, Lina, with a big grin on her face, would dash right out into the water, shouting, "Swim! Swim! Go swim, Mama!" And

I, unable to control the smile that spread from ear to ear on my own face, would throw off my jacket and hat and shoes and jump in after her, aware that even though her intention to swim was wholehearted, my little adventurous girl had yet to learn how, and lacked the fear that kept most other children at a safe distance from deeper water and higher waves. Lina would be drenched by one such wave, much larger than her own tiny but muscular little body, come up for air as it settled, spit and laugh and scream, "More, more!" Her life-affirming, go-getter attitude was inspirational to me. It was so much healthier than the attitude of many fearful, suspicious fellow beings, and yet, in our day-to-day life, her bold-ness was almost impossible to handle. As the cold water during the winter months quickly became too intense for me to handle, I had to drag a screaming and kicking Lina out of the water, throw her up on my shoulders, and run to our car. Was it worth it? Yes it was. And I quickly learned to keep extra clothes in the back of the car for both of us. Why did the ice-cold water not bother Lina? Her sensory receptors didn't seem to register input as effectively as most of us. In order for her to feel what most of us feel, she had to take everything to its ultimate edge. Living with Lina was to live a life right at that edge. It meant becoming familiar with one's own breaking point as well. It meant coming very close, on a daily basis, to what one traditionally believes one cannot handle.

Sometimes I didn't just come up toward my own edge but I came tumbling down the steep hill beyond. One night after a long, exhausting day with Lina, she was as hyperactive as she'd ever been. For hours, she'd been jumping around the bedroom, laughing and shouting, throwing herself on me (I had moved Elsa into a different bedroom right after she, against all odds, had fallen asleep in the midst of all the commotion), until I heard myself lose my cool. I hollered at her to stop and then ran away from her down the stairs to the living room in huge, desperate steps. I took the basement stairs in leaping steps and hid there with my anger and despair, crying desperately into a pillow on the floor. Everything was quiet for a moment. I just sat there on the ugly dark green basement carpet witnessing my own fear of throwing my little girl out the window. I called Anki, crying on the phone about my own limitations, the injustice I had just committed to Lina by screaming at her, and the injustice of what I felt were inhumane expectations of me to handle something that seemed so impossible. I heard Lina coming after me down the stairs and, unable to face her, I fled out the door to the dark backyard. There I sat, sobbing into the phone with my loving friend just listening and understanding without a trace of judgment, reminding me how well I handled the situation most of the time and how I had to stop expecting that I would always be able to do it perfectly. It was such a relief to admit that all I wanted to do in that moment was to give up, get into my car, and drive away. Away from my daughter's relentless hyperactivity, away from the impossible, away from having to face what I couldn't do, away from having to try to find ways to negotiate everything with Tony, away from the island with all the strangers who seemed so impossible to get to know, and away from my own judgment of myself. Being allowed to say it to someone who was 100 percent capable of appreciating my experience, and who communicated that understanding as effectively as Anki did in that miserable moment, made it easier to go back into the house, take Lina's hand, and walk up the stairs and try again.

The best interactions consistently happened in the playroom. There was the morning when we were listening to a song from a CD called *Music Together* about going to grandma's house to pick cherries. While we were singing along together, Lina was piggy-back riding, and I jumped around with her while we both maintained eye contact through the mirror. Lina laughed and squealed and was intensively connected to me in that moment. When the song was over, I told her how much I loved her and how happy I was to be with her. With her face closely pressed against mine, she smiled and said, "I love you," and then kissed me. Tears instantly came to my eyes. I couldn't remember when I had last heard those words from my daughter. It was almost hard to register. I felt so happy and peaceful. We were going in the right direction. I wasn't lost anymore. I knew what to do. I knew something about how I could help my daughter. She would come back to us.

It was a Wednesday morning in early September when Lina suddenly, out of the blue, said something that reinforced the notion of the usefulness of our time in the playroom in a way that I had never witnessed before. For Christmas the previous year, Anki had sent us porcelain cups, one to Lina and one to Elsa, each with a picture of their friends Ellen and Alfred. This morning up in the playroom, Lina initiated an unusually reflective dialogue about these "nice cups." I asked Lina, "Who is it on the cups?" While only rarely responding to questions, Lina, this time, simply said, "Ellen och Alfred" (Ellen and Alfred). Then she added, "Nice cups, they are such nice cups!" Moved and excited, I hugged my daughter and said, "I love it when you're telling me things."

"Yes," said Lina, "but it's so hard sometimes."

"Yes, baby, it is, but you are doing really well!" I told her. Encouraged and still in my arms, Lina again reflected on the cups, "Dom ar sa fina koppar!" (They are such nice cups!) And then, to my ongoing amazement, she continued, "and Ellen and Lina had such nice hair and nice dresses." While it had been Ellen and

Alfred's pictures on the cups, Lina was inspired by this thoughtful gift, and had continued to associate from her friendship with Ellen, describing another memorable moment of being dressed up with her friend. Tears now streamed down my face as I hugged and kissed my little heroine. You are in the desert and someone offers a bottle of cold water. You see the sun rise after you thought the sun would never rise again. When you hold your newborn baby in your arms for the very first time. That was what I felt hearing those beautiful words from my daughter's mouth.

I started to notice the difference in Lina's behavior between days when we had a lot of time in the playroom and the days that we didn't. She was much more hyperactive and out of touch on the days when we hadn't had the chance to be together in that intense, focused way up in the playroom. Overall, she had almost stopped biting completely. As everyone involved in autism will know, it is very difficult, maybe impossible, to know the causes involved in both the progression and subsiding of the symptoms. I consciously decided to stop wasting my time obsessing about those unconquerable questions and felt satisfied knowing that Tony and I, to the best of our ability, had tried to approach Lina's condition from as many angles as possible. It was clear that symbolic thinking and pretend play was almost exclusively evident in the playroom. After I eliminated Play-Doh because Lina ate it and it contained the gluten for which we now were on a vigilant lookout, Lina used clay for most of her pretend play. She pretended to make scones, pears, pancakes, and ice cream. She made cinnamon buns, chicken soup, and birthday cakes. We made meatballs and pizza and cheese sandwiches and sliced ham. Everything that Lina wanted to eat, but couldn't because of her diet, materialized in the clay. There was no end to the food games. And I felt so happy and at peace with being in there with my little girl, cooking up a storm, every day being a new opportunity to recapture lost ground and to find territories that neither Lina nor I had ever visited before. Up there, yesterday and tomorrow paled in comparison to the potential miracles that might come out of Lina's eyes and language. And when Janet and Jackie and Maryanne and Susan had their chance to drop their lives and just be with Lina, they spontaneously expressed a similar sense of wonder and personal development.

And Elsa and I, for the first time in the very difficult year and a half that had passed, had new opportunities to find each other and play and cook and read books and talk without the constant interruption of Lina climbing the cupboards, hunting for food, or eating the crayons or dumping all of our shampoo in the toilet. Elsa loved that time, when we could do whatever we wanted without worries that something would fall apart. With this opportunity, it became painfully obvious how complicated life already was for my little two-and-a-half-year-old. Since that past spring, Lina had been going to see Chrystal, a speech therapist, and Theresa, an occupational therapist, who teamed up with Chrystal and worked in the same office. Elsa really counted on those two and three forty-five-minute sessions per week in the speech and occupational therapist's office, where she and I could read books and play with the toys in the waiting room.

Chrystal, with her warm, optimistic, and engaging personality, and Theresa, with her thoughtful, innovative approach to occupational therapy, were wonderful to Lina. But even Chrystal and Theresa agreed that increasing one-on-one time in the playroom was where our resources would be best spent. We decided to stop the speech and OT with Chrystal and Theresa and utilize them more as consultants, whenever I needed them to help me figure something out from working with Lina in the playroom. I began training new people to work with Lina in the playroom.

The Son-Rise Program, the inspiration behind the playroom, holds seminars for families to support and inspire parents, relatives, friends, and volunteers to do intensive, one-on-one work with their children in the playroom. I convinced Tony to come with me and spend a week in a lodge near the Option Institute in Sheffield, Massachusetts, while I spent most of the days at the institute, processing and learning about how to provide the most effective support and inspiration to Lina and facilitate her way back to us. The instructors and teachers were wonderful and helped me think about everything from training new people in the playroom to how to inspire language in Lina to how to become an irresistible fellow human being to my daughter, even on days when she preferred to be left alone rather than interacting and engaging with me.

Still, the most significant inspiration of that week in Massachusetts was all the other parents. Over lunches and coffee breaks and during discussions in the cozy conference room, we shared our tears and triumphs, fears and visions for our children with each other. I met Magnus, a red-headed, very Viking-looking Swede who, amazingly, lived a couple of miles away from the tiny little village where I myself grew up. His humble and yet bold and irrefutable insistence on saving his six-year-old daughter from disappearing from him, his wife, and their four-year-old daughter, moved me. He came all the way from Sweden, spending his nights sweating about how his wife would make out alone in the house with a daughter who wouldn't sleep, and his days, quietly focused and open, listening to every word anyone uttered that could help him in the quest to reach his little girl.

There was the shy woman, who struggled with her own doubts about her ability to build a better relationship with her teenage son. She often stayed close by my side, hoping for words of encouragement, struggling to share her story and mustering up all the courage she could grab hold of to ask if we could exchange email addresses and keep in touch after the week had passed. There was the English couple with the warm, insightful husband and the passionate, intelligent wife who moved closer and closer together in their learning and shared experience. They gave each other so much room to make their own individual observations, free from the interpretation of the other, and yet they were so closely knit together, like two horses pulling the same carriage, effectively, rapidly, in the same direction.

The week was filled with encouraging handshakes, hearty embraces, shared tears and laughter, and stories of our children finding or recapturing new words. There were stories and tears about moments of shame and hopelessness, when parental patience was exploited to the maximum by hyperactive children and everything was falling apart, in anger and desperation. There was forgiveness and love, and faith in each others' ability to resolve unsolvable problems. We laughed at all the compromises involved in living with children whose nervous systems have lost all predictability. We giggled at all the funny things one says under pressure and made fun of the outrageous reactions from people who didn't know what it was like to live in the world of autism.

Since our separation, Tony and I had never had such a great connection as during this week. Jackie and Valerie, for a couple of days each, assisted Tony in making the days agreeable while I was away on training. We spent the evenings eating Chinese food in nearby Great Barrington. In the mornings, I sent Tony to the main house of the hotel for breakfast and a couple of moments of peace before another intense day. Late nights, after both girls fell asleep, Tony and I would stay up in the little kitchen next to my and the girls' bedroom, celebrating Son-Rise, Lina, and Elsa, as well as our own improved connection. I had my peppermint tea. Tony had his chamomile tea. And both of us, faithful to a long marital tradition, had our nightly ice cream pints. Yes, one full pint each, without any problem. People sometimes ask me how I can eat the impressive quantity of food that I do without becoming massively obese. Others look at Tony's finely toned arms and legs and wonder how they can become members of the same gym he belongs to. An hour with Lina would help them understand. It's not the miracle work of some personal trainer or secret diet. It is the constant movement and very physical engagement in the latest whereabouts of a little girl who never stops.

Back home again, the work with Lina in the playroom continued. Our team of dynamic women continued working with Lina upstairs whenever I needed to be elsewhere. Lina, with her open spirit and loving heart, accepted them all. Now and then, we met as a group to discuss our work with Lina, observe her progress, and think through potential obstacles to her learning new levels of relatedness and expressiveness. Jackie, with her innovativeness; Valerie, with her down-to-earth, all-accepting attitude; Susan, with her humor and spunk; Janet, with her humble, loving presence; and Maryanne, with her subtle consideration and peacefulness, were all part of the team. They all fell in love with Lina in their own way and none of them failed to understand that this wasn't a process to cure Lina. This was a mutually beneficial journey where the main goal was to find a way to get to know Lina and ourselves, share our world with Lina and invite her to share her world with us. I never told anyone that directly. It was just abundantly clear to everyone that here was a person with an unusually warm heart, an unusually generous spirit, a young person, someone who had lost the ability or the will to talk and access words, but still, a person who would be both teacher and student to anyone who would be willing and lucky enough to get to know her. That was the basic premise.

Lina made a lot of strides, verbally as well as in terms of relatedness and more calmness. It still wasn't calm. And every night after my girls went to sleep, I took deep breaths in amazement that that particular day had passed. I still chased my little girl around the house from early morning to late at night. And I felt very alone and overwhelmed by the daily responsibility of making sure Lina wasn't run over by a car or eating toothpaste and crayons and that Elsa was allowed some kind of reasonable childhood in the midst of all the madness. I had to face myself, compromise, and fail many times a day. I didn't feel victorious and self-assured. I understood that I had to give my life over to a higher power. I didn't want to. But I had to.

One night I woke up to a big bang, as though something big had fallen on the house. I know this sounds strange, but I was simply too tired to look out the window. "Whatever it is, I'll deal with it tomorrow," I thought and went back to sleep. Then I had a nightmare. I dreamed that a tree had fallen on our house and destroyed my kitchen. The walls surrounding the kitchen were in ruins and the kitchen demolished. I spent a big portion of the dream trying to find electricians and carpenters who could fix our kitchen. It didn't go well. I woke up the next morning, sweating, looked out the window, and saw that the main branch of the huge oak tree in our yard had broken in the wind and fallen onto the house, just on the right side of our bedroom window. It had snapped the wires so we had lost our cable Internet connection. But my kitchen was intact.

The next night, I was on the phone with Anki, laughing and joking about the tree being a symbolic God's arm putting a curse on me and my life, eternally testing and pushing my limits to see when I would snap. Just as Anki and I were laughing about this, Elsa, who had been sleeping behind me, pressed up against my back for comfort, woke up and said, "Mama, there are many trees that didn't fall on our house." Her comment became one of the most precious reminders in my life. Clearly, my little angel was right. Only my very egocentrist perspective prevented me from seeing beyond the hardship to all the beauty of our current life, all the preciousness and bliss. The very fact that Elsa was lying there, close to me and so comfortable just being there. Lina, with all her mystery and love. Anki. The ocean a couple of miles from our house. The rest of the beautiful tree outside our house, still capable of holding two swings and one swinging ladder from its sturdy branches. The list was endless.

There were many moments and days of joy and bliss on this beautiful island. Together with Michael and Lauren and their four kids, we leased Sunny, a chestnut-colored large pony, at a gorgeous stable built with old-fashioned British architecture and surrounded by acres and acres of breathtaking meadows and hills just next to the ocean. Lauren, together with her older children, Kevin, Alicia, and Burke, took care of Sunny and rode him three days a week. Lina and Elsa had wonderful opportunities to ride Sunny on the weekends. I would ride with them, sometimes bareback and sometimes with a saddle, with Lina or Elsa in my lap in front of me. Lauren would walk next to us, to prevent Sunny from turning around and trotting back to his beloved stable. Horseback riding is a well-known resource in autism circles. Lina enjoyed the motion of the horse and sitting there, tightly pressed up against me right behind her. She would stay on for up to twenty minutes at a time before she started to try to throw herself toward the ground. With Lina, trying to convince her of something she didn't want to do was very close to futile. As soon as she was done, she was done, and it was only a matter of getting her to land on the ground without injuries. Lauren's kids would chase her around while Elsa had her chance to ride with Mama.

Now and then, we would all have big family gatherings out there on one of the meadows after such rides. Other times we would go to one of the beaches. We would bring meat and corn on the cob and fruit and chips and Tony and I would alternate running after Lina, who loved to search around for berries, rotten apples, and anything else she could potentially put in her mouth. Not infrequently, if we were in the presence of the ocean or the fresh air or wide open spaces, Tony and I would relax enough to find our way back to our old ways of kidding around, mocking each others' quirks, Tony trying to chase me down and me sprinting away from him, startling or amusing other picnickers in the area. We would fight over morsels of food and Tony and Michael would complain about the way my portions didn't match my size while I would insist that it was a matter of variations in metabolism. Our children would look at us with big eyes and relax. This seemed like things used to be, Mama and Papa teasing each other and having fun, not the tense, withholding, mutual discontent they had so often witnessed in the past three years.

CHAPTER FIVE

Going Back Home

In spite of such golden moments, in spite of the ocean than never failed to entice with its endless, glittering, ever-changing vitality and beauty, one day at the end of the summer, a beach experience brought ideas of moving back to New York City closer to the surface. Lina, Elsa, and I were on a very crowded beach one sunny Sunday afternoon. There was a mother on the beach, screaming at me to control my children. Lina had taken a bucket from her daughter as her daughter played in the surf and had also splashed water, some of it landing on this mother's little girl. Indignant and furious, the mother came from her seated position in the sand to remove her daughter. Her daughter hadn't objected to the splashing and didn't seem to care about the bucket, but that didn't seem to have much impact on her mother. With dirty looks in our direction and muttering disapproval between tight lips, she dragged her daughter out of the water. Continuing to chase my unruly daughter down the beach, I thought about this ongoing situation. People in a place without much diversity have very little opportunity and emotional resources to welcome and accept someone like Lina. This is an island where most people know everybody else. And yet, very few people seem interested in getting to know someone as unusual and intense as Lina. Later, as Lina ran back out into the water, the little girl's father, who had witnessed the water-bucket situation, took his daughter by the hand and led her back out into the water, demonstratively walking next to Lina and smiling apologetically. I smiled back and felt tears filling up my eyes, as always happens when someone shows understanding and compassion where previously only judgment and fear could be found.

A few minutes afterward, Tony came to the beach to take the girls for the rest of the afternoon. He found me sitting with Lina and Elsa in the sand with an empty, tired look on my face. "Tony, have you ever thought about moving back to the city?"

"All the time," he replied.

Diversity and tolerance, a better public school system for children with special needs, homesickness, and isolation were all factors that spoke for a return to New York City. Also, we were losing some of our wonderful babysitters and playroom helpers. Jackie and Maryanne were graduating and moving to the mainland. Janet's husband had been reassigned to a different city. Time after time, both Tony and I found ourselves making appointments with babysitters who never showed up. Furthermore, Tony's family—his parents Nick and Mari, his brother Charlie, and his sister Jennifer, her husband Steve, and their two kids were all in New York. Elsa was becoming big enough to go with her grandparents for lunch and her cousin Finn, just a few years older, was a perfect companion for Elsa. With him as well as with other boy playmates, Elsa connected with a more daring, wild side of herself, which was important for Elsa who often overcompensated for Lina's hyperactivity and lack of impulse control by being extra cautious and compliant. And while Nick and Mari did not have the energy to chase after Lina, Grandma Mari seemed to have a special place in Lina's heart. Lina would come up to her and check out her face and wonderful, soft, curly hair, and smile.

One day, as Valerie (who always showed up when she said she would) and I were unpacking the car and bringing the girls back into the house, I told her about our plans to move back to New York. Then I said, almost on an impulse, "Maybe you want to come with us?" Valerie smiled and said, "Funny you should ask, since lately I've been thinking about leaving Newport and wouldn't mind living in New York for some time." There wasn't much discussion. Somehow it seemed like the most natural thing in the world that Valerie would come with us. She was so easy to be around and capable of handling whatever came her way. She was exactly what we needed and became a kind of transitional link for both Lina and Elsa between life in Newport and our new-old life in New York City.

It took us a few months after this realization to prepare for the move back. By mid-December, and hundreds of productive, intriguing, and fun-filled playroom hours later, we packed up and left. During one of my work trips to the city, after a long day of sessions with my clients downtown, I walked into an apartment on the Upper West Side at eight thirty, accompanied by one of the few agents that were willing to show places that late on a Friday night. I saw our new home. The place was dark and messy and unrenovated and a neighbor downstairs claimed that it was no longer on the market since he had already made a deal for it with the owner and wanted to show me *his* place instead. But I had already seen the light. It was perfect. It had one room with windows facing both north and east that we would use as a playroom for our continued work with Lina. There we could do all the same things we had done in our upstairs playroom in Newport, but with the happy and grounding feeling of being at the center of the world. The dining room area could be closed off from the living room by replacing doors that had been there many years previously, affording me a space that I could utilize as a home office and, initially, allowing Valerie a place to put her bed and a space to stay until she found her own. The apartment was a block away from Fairway, the most incredible market with absolutely everything a household might need and with an additional upstairs health-food section that supports all of the special diet needs a family with a child with autism might require. I walked out of the apartment sure that this would be our next home.

Driving in the car with Valerie, Elsa, and Lina, was one of the most joyous and happy trips we had ever taken. Leaving Newport and moving back to New York City felt like the most natural, logical, and reasonable thing in the world. All four of us were singing along loudly with Akon's "Mama Africa" (Lina's favorite), and Van Morrison's "Days Like This" for most of the way. Coming down the West Side Highway, passing the George

Washington Bridge, and driving along the Hudson River, I felt the warm feeling of homecoming. Life was good. The isolated life on an island where most people had never met a girl as active and unpredictable as Lina was over.

Of course, Tony and I still watched Lina's adjustment to our new situation with apprehension. We had already put her through so many changes, now this! But we had made every move in good faith and thoroughly believed that New York City, after all, was the best option for all of us. We arrived on December 12 and by the next day, Lina was already working with me and Valerie in the playroom. In my notebook, I wrote:

> *Lina is dealing with the move beyond expectation. While some increasing stimming (self-stimulatory behavior), clapping hands, making "mmmm" sounds, watching own hands more and using repetitive phrases and more incoherent language, she has been relatively calm, actually calmer than in Newport! Maybe related to new theanine supplement or the HTP5 that Dr. Lynch had recommended for her but it could also be the calm before the storm or a kind of shock of the move. Or, it could be that she, like Tony and I, is also experiencing a kind of relief of being back home in New York. Her eye contact, mood, and relating are already improving and she is well settled in the playroom, working with me and Valerie intermittently. Today, we had an amazing session.*

A week into our new living situation, Lina seemed more involved and interactive than she had been for many months. In a progress note from December 19, I noted her rapid adjustment:

Working with stickers mostly. Lina is very related in a low-keyed way. Requests very coherent and with splendid eye contact. Dancing today was amazing. Lina came up with one dance move and/or game after the other. Happy and relaxed mood. Flexible about things we didn't have and accepting of alternatives. Little or no stimming and instead sustained involvement and active interest in our interaction. Lovely session. Lots of singing and some games were inspired by songs like "This Is the Way We Bake our Bread" (Swedish version). Lina initiated many songs and movements herself.

It was so beautiful to be back in New York. And Lina and Elsa and Valerie and I enjoyed our new life together. In the mornings, Lina and Elsa and I came into the kitchen next to the former dining room that now was my office and Valerie's bedroom for our breakfast pancakes. With me focused on the pancakes, the girls would amuse themselves by jumping on Valerie in her big, comfortable bed. Valerie, who is one of the most patient, well-adjusted young individuals I have had the chance to get to know, would just smile, turn the other way, and keep on sleeping. Lina would stay there until the pancakes were done, having made her way under the blanket next to Valerie, singing and talking to herself. Elsa would stand next to my desk, drawing and playing with her dolls and animals, making up elaborate stories about all of their dramatic adventures.

Apart from finding ways to expand our interactions with Lina, one important component of our work with her in the playroom was to reestablish her capacity and joy for pretend play. This, as the most important foundation for symbolic thinking and subsequent reading and writing and expressing more abstract matters, was not easy. Lina operated, and still does, on a very concrete level. Abstract thinking is for the most part out of her reach. Lina's participation in any kind of pretend play, if only for brief moments, was always celebrated. After a couple of weeks in our new home, Lina accepted that one of her teddy bears desperately wanted some of her blueberries. Lina, who has always been generous, gave him three, placing them in his paws, and ate the rest herself. I teased her about the fact that she only volunteered three blueberries. She smiled. I smiled, too. This was a very important symbolic gesture.

Only a couple of weeks into our return to New York City, Lina's expressive language as well as emotional availability and transparency were as strong as they had been since all that had gone into hiding, a year and a half earlier. Right before Christmas, Valerie had the following session with Lina.

> She was mad at me, even bit my wrist pretty hard at one point. . . . She wanted more stickers. She was actually very angry with me about it when she bit me though I think she felt really bad because she sat quietly on her knees with her hands at her mouth and kept glancing at me with guilty/ sorry eyes. After that she wanted to be carried and we put on "Single Ladies" and it cheered her right up. We sat on the ball (she asked in a full sentence to sit on the blue "balloon" ball). Tons of eye contact and interaction that at last set our moods straight. At the end, we popped some more balloons. The last one we did popped so loud and Lina said on her very own, "It's a bursting balloon."

In a session a couple of days later, as Lina and I had been cutting out pictures from various magazines, Lina, unprompted, commented, "It's the countryside." As we were ending that session, Lina smiled and hugged me and said, "I feel great!" Lina's increasing emotional expressiveness also led to more deliberate demonstration of affection. In one of Valerie's sessions, Lina gives her the full treatment:

> *At the very end of our time Lina got on my back while we danced to hip-hop in the mirror. She was just calmly lying there with no expression on her face and of course here I was all wide-eyed, smiling big. So I said, "Lina, can you give me a great big smile?" and she gave me a great big kiss on my cheek and then she proceeded to turn my head and gave me another great big peck on the lips. I said, "Well, thank you, Lina, for the kisses; they were so very nice, but I still would love to see a great big wonderful Lina smile." She gave me a kiss on my cheek and then turned and looked at me through the mirror and just started laughing. It was great!*

Lina was on her way. Everyone around her was excited about Lina's new involvement and expressiveness. It was so good to be back in New York and to see that she, like her little sister who was thrilled about all the new playgrounds, filled with potential new playmates, was responding well to this change. And yet, this winter, for me, was also marked by my mother's progressing cancer. I ended Lina's first playroom notebook with the following letter to Lina:

> *Lina,*
> *This book describes the most interesting journey a mother can take with her child. You made it so. And Valerie, Janet,*

Marion, Susan, Jackie, Maryanne, and I learned a lot about
you and even more about ourselves. Your grandmother is
dying. But you are coming back to us. We are really playing
together now, and I appreciate every second of the time we
are together. Thank you, Lina.
   Love,
   Your Mother.

In my own journal, in January of 2009, I tried to process the
fact that my mother had just told me that she would rather I
come to her funeral than be next to her at her deathbed. I understood this request on multiple levels but will elaborate on the part
of it that relates to Lina. Like me, my mother likes order. Having
Lina around, inevitably, eliminates order. My mother knew that
I would not travel anywhere without my daughters. My feelings
about my mother's request came out in a letter to Lina. This letter
I would never send to my daughter. It was really a letter to myself:

I'm going to give you something that I don't have. I'm giving
it to you because from my limited, maternal perspective, I
need to give it. It's a promise. I promise you, Lina, that I
won't die until you can live your life happily without me.
Your grandmother is dying. I'm not afraid of her dying. I can
live my life happily without her. But I'm afraid of not being
by her side when she dies. Does she not want me to come
because of you, Lina? Maybe it's a consequence of our last
summer's visit to Sweden when you climbed on the coun-
tertops in her kitchen in your neverending search for food,
destroyed two doors [somehow she managed to get the doors
off their hinges and break them!], ripped the pages out of her
books, and pulled the leaves off of her plants?

Lina, I know you didn't do any of it maliciously. Your world is different than mine. Everyone—from the stranger on Broadway who skeptically watches your loud singing and restless running in and out of stores touching everything you see, to close friends and relatives who know you well—wants you to accept the premises of their world. I understand that. I've wanted the same thing for you. Very few people in your life have been willing to move fully into your experience. From what I have understood, everything, past and present, visual and auditory, material and concrete as well as abstract, is exploding against your senses with lightning speed. Sometimes, destroying some of these things or putting them in your mouth may be the only way you have to attain some kind of understanding of their nature. Or it may be your way of forcing things around you to slow down. Maybe it's also the most effective way for you to connect and interact with your environment. All I know is that it's fruitless to punish or blame you for the things that you do in your world just because it's unacceptable and inconvenient or considered destructive in mine.

Your sweetness and affection, your soft arms around my neck, your cheek pressed tightly against mine, as we listen and laugh to Norah Jones and Dolly Parton's duet "Creepin' in" or Akon's song about a girl who is like "fire burning on the dance floor," compensates for all the confusion I feel about your life experience being so different from mine. My relentless desire to understand you will have to do as the bridge between our different realities. I hope you can feel that what makes us react so differently can be an intriguing exploration. I feel that way now, most of the time. It took me a while to get there.

My last few phone conversations with my mother became increasingly incoherent. She was so tired and weak, it was hard for her to express herself in words. Then one day, as Elsa and I were sitting at Utopia, our favorite diner, eating scrambled eggs and croissants on our weekly Monday lunch date, my brother Staffan called. As I put down the phone, my little girl looked at me:

"Mama, why are you crying?"

I told Elsa about her grandmother moving on. We were sitting there, tears sliding down both our cheeks, talking about how, even if Grandma was ready to die, ready to move on, we would miss her as she was in this life.

A couple weeks later, Lina and Elsa and Valerie and I were on an airplane to Sweden. My father picked us up at the airport, smiling and acting as if nothing had happened. No tears, no disbelief, no signs of shock, no nothing. I looked at my father and wondered how it was possible that I could have grown up in the same household as him and yet know so little about him. Did Lina and my father have similar struggles to remain present and communicative in this world? Or was it Lina and her artistic paternal grandmother, whose lap Lina always crept up in as soon as she showed up, who had something in common? Or maybe she got it from me? From second grade through fourth grade, my teachers were concerned that I spent most of my time daydreaming, not engaged in the social world around me. In the classroom, I used to disappear into my own thoughts while gazing out the window, missing everything my teachers said. During recess, I would stand leaning on the pink stone wall of the main school building, looking without seeing the other kids running around. I would run my hand over the rough surface of the wall, deep in thought. Being back in Sweden always brought that old surreal feeling back. Being there without really being there. Did I pass that on to my wonderful little girl? But Lina, when she smiles and really looks and engages with someone, even if she doesn't utter a single word, can be so present and direct that people sometimes feel uneasy and put on the spot. Other times, she disappears.

As during our last visit to Sweden, after a few initial days of being overstimulated, Lina did wonderfully. From day one, we set up a playroom and Valerie and I took turns being in there with Lina, singing, playing with clay, cutting up magazines, and talking about books and picture albums just like we did in New York. When Lina was three, one of her favorite books was about a Native American girl named Leelanau, who goes off to live in the spirit world. In one of those sessions, Lina made the connection between Leelanau's spirit world and her grandmother's death, saying that "Grandma went to the spirit world." "Mmm," I said, "it was her time to go. She was ready." Lina didn't seem to have any trouble accepting her grandmother's disappearance to the spirit world. Elsa, on the other hand, had much more anxiety about her grandmother's death and the possibility of me disappearing just like Grandma. At the funeral, which Lina didn't attend since her presence would have turned a peaceful event in remembrance of my mother into a disorderly situation where grief and tears would have been displaced by an astonishing event featuring an almost six-year-old little girl with thick, blond, curly hair and an unstoppable energy level. The churchgoers, my mother's relatives and friends, would have forgotten all about my mother. Lina would have stolen my mother's last show. I contemplated this scenario, tempted by my own curiosity about people's reactions to Lina's unconventional, intense presence in a situation that insists upon order and stillness, but recognized that this probably wouldn't have been what my mother wanted. Elsa, though, in the midst of the ceremony, made her own little mark on the event when, just before everyone was to walk up to the coffin to say their goodbyes to my mother, she said in a loud voice: "Grandma isn't really dead!" I knew what she meant and I share her belief, but the timing of this insight could have been better. Or maybe not. Eventually, the funeral turned into a wonderful celebration of my mother's passionate, high-energy, headstrong, and always humorous existence in this life. Lina and Elsa and Valerie and I left Sweden a week later with a good feeling of mission completed, eager to be back in New York.

Lina, unlike many children with autism, often seemed to thrive on change. Sometimes I think boredom is her greatest challenge. Given her difficulties with symbolic thinking and pretend play, she has a hard time having fun. Fun becomes pushing people's buttons, living on the edge, making people's faces turn red and distorted when they think she has gone too far and don't know how to make her stop whatever it is she is doing. Unlike with regular kids, it doesn't feel okay to get mad at Lina. Even when she throws scissors and spoons out the window and chews on our favorite CDs or pulls my shirt up all the way to my throat in the middle of crowded Broadway, I know she doesn't have a mean bone in her body. She likes intensity. She desperately seeks sensory input and is very interested in closeness with people around her but she doesn't know how to engage. For her, seeing people flustered is a confirmation of such engagement. When someone chases her around, Lina is present for the chase and not at risk of disappearing into her own, quiet, isolated world.

Life with Lina is great Zen training. It is an incredible opportunity to learn about one's own edge, one's own panic and frustration, one's own rigid, preconceived notions of how things should be. Lina mentally turns you upside down, forcing you to see everything from a completely different angle from the moment she comes out of her early morning, cuddly state of drowsiness, until she reluctantly closes her eyes in the late evening, after hours of curtain pulling, jumping around the bed, and making innumerable trips to the bathroom, each time squeezing out a little bit more pee to defend her credibility.

In many ways, when carefully balanced with plenty of one-on-one time in the playroom, New York City and the Upper West Side were perfect for Lina. New Yorkers have seen it all. Lina didn't shock and annoy people the same way as she did in Newport. For a mother who constantly had to apologize for her daughter's inability to control her impulses, for snatching other people's snacks, running up the slide the wrong way, puncturing other children's water balloons, it was deeply comforting to have another parent say, "It's okay, I understand." It kept the feeling of impending catastrophe at bay.

CHAPTER SIX

Finding School

During the spring and summer of 2009, our days were structured around play sessions and breaks. After breakfast, Lina and I had our first two hours in the playroom. Then Valerie and Lina had another two-hour session before lunch break. After lunch, Lina and I went back to the playroom and worked a little more before we all got ready to go outside. After some park time, Elsa and I would hang out and make dinner while Valerie and Lina had the day's last play session. We only rarely changed around our daily rhythm and all benefited from that clarity of the task at hand. Now and then, someone else came in to take Valerie's sessions to give her a break.

In the playroom notebook, we all reported Lina's most outstanding verbalizations:

"Mama, make a heart!" (Lina is asking me to make a heart out of clay.)

"You're ready for lunch!" (Without any prompting, Lina is telling Valerie that she, Lina, is ready for lunch.)

"Remember driving far into the night?" (Lina was taking a break in her bouncing on the trampoline, looked right at me, and recalled this event that took place as we drove late evening to Massachusetts to attend the Son-Rise program. Lina had been awake the whole time and loved sitting in her car seat with me next to her, listening to music, chatting, and looking at the world passing by the car window.)

One morning, as Lina was eating her pancake with all the supplements mixed in with some sugar-free jam on top, I asked Lina, "What should we do today?"

"Play!" she responded with an intention and enthusiasm that almost brought joyful tears to my eyes.

As Lina's conversations and interactions in the playroom developed, her intention solidified. She knew what she wanted, and as the playroom was full of possibility and very little limitation, she seemed to feel increasingly motivated to find the words that she needed to make her wishes come true. We did a lot of celebration of Lina in the playroom. Lina loved this attention. And it was genuine. Every day Valerie and I, as well as Elsa, noted more progress in Lina's verbalizations and pretend play. And she showed more initiative in relating to everyone around her. And we had fun. We came up with some really crazy dance moves in the playroom. We did obstacle courses. We covered ourselves and each other in finger-paints. We cracked nuts until nutshells covered the entire playroom floor. We blew balloons until our faces were purple and popped them until our ears went numb. We did endless tickle and chase games until Lina teared up from pure laughter.

Slowly, Lina and Elsa began to find little ways to converse and interact. One morning, as Lina and Elsa and I were lying around on our futons, Elsa was talking, saying something about Mr. Nobody. Lina leaned forward toward Elsa, looked directly at her, smiled, and said, "Mr. Nobody!" Elsa just stared at her, then looked at me with a classic "Wow-did-you-see-and-hear-that?!" look. I kissed both my girls and thought about the possibility that one day they would be able to really play together, and talk, and maybe even share each other's secrets, or complain about me and Tony, or pretend that they were on a special mission to the moon or that they were good fairies saving the world together.

Gradually, Lina began to get a better sense of how to pretend. Blown-up balloons could be giant berries and ice-cream cones and the punctured ones could become a fried egg. One of our blankets could become a boat where Lina and Elsa could sit as I would drag it along the apartment, pretending to take them to Sweden to visit Paulina and Felicia and Alicia (their cousins) and back again since Papa missed you soooo much.

Being outside only rarely allowed for pretend play opportunities. Lina was too busy searching for discarded wads of chewing gum on the ground. One never has such a clear sense of how vast the chewing gum spitting tradition is until one has a child who loves to pick chewed-up pieces from the ground and put them in her mouth. Nothing helped. Preventing her didn't help. Ignoring it didn't help. Giving her consequences for chewing on other people's gum didn't help. Giving Lina her own chewing gum didn't help—she just spit it out as soon as she saw another wad, flattened out on the ground. Lina's restricted diet made forbidden foods a tantalizing treasure. When we took Lina to a place in Central Park where a man with funny, pink hair was letting kids play his drums and flutes and maracas, Lina was much more interested in the nearby ice-cream stand. She figured if she tore down the salesman's ice-cream sign, she might find the real stuff. The man asked me if I wanted to buy some. "No thanks," I said and apologized for Lina's transgression. The man smiled, as if to seduce me into giving in to my child's desire for this sugar-packed casein that would send her tripping. He asked me again. "No," I replied sternly, "and don't ask me again." Lina went back to trying to tear up his ice-cream sign but the man, in spite of my surliness, maintained his patience with Lina's hands-on interest in his ice-cream sign. I shrugged and looked at him. We both smiled. Our conflict of interest didn't prevent us from a moment of mutual understanding. That's what I love about New York. That evening, before going to bed, Lina took my face in her hands and looked straight into my eyes, smiling warmly and with the kind of openness that can move mountains. That's what I love about Lina. That's what everyone loves about Lina.

This classic Lina smile got her forgiven for a lot of her transgressions. Lina had found a new way of testing her Papa's patience. She was at his new apartment not far from ours. Lina was sitting on top of his desk, banging his keyboard with her fists. Now and then she stopped, glancing over at Tony with a devilish look on her face. Then she returned to her newfound project and, with accelerated delight, banged harder. Finding the joy and the ability to let go within himself, Tony decided that if need be he could buy a new keyboard for fifty dollars, but if he didn't take the chance to capture that little devilish look and pure delight on his daughter's face with a camera, the moment would be gone forever.

The more playroom time Lina got, the less she engaged with people by testing their limits. Now and then, Elsa was invited to play with Lina and me or Valerie in the playroom. We would sit by the little table and work with clay together, or blow up balloons, one to Lina, the other to Elsa. Sometimes we would put on music and all bounce on the bouncing ball together, Lina in my lap, or Valerie's, and Elsa hanging onto our backs. Lina seemed more aware of Elsa as a person of potential. She would listen to one of Elsa's elaborate stories about princesses and crocodiles and pirate ships and smile. She would share her food with her little sister like a real champion. Even the things she really loved, like grapes and blueberries, she would readily hand over whenever her little sister requested it.

We also invited Eila, one of Lina's friends from before autism, to play with us in the playroom, bouncing away to Akon and Stevie Wonder, blowing bubbles or jumping on the trampoline or chasing each other around the room for crazy-making tickles. Lina and Eila had the kind of soul connection that Lina only developed with a handful of her closest friends. Very few things compare to seeing Lina laughing and bouncing on the trampoline with this beautiful little girl.

Ellen, Lina's very first real girlfriend, was visiting New York with her father, who continued to work for UNICEF even after the family had moved back to Stockholm. One day Ellen and Lina and Elsa and Valerie and I had a popcorn and fruit-salad party in the playroom. It started out civilized, with all of us sitting around on the soft mat on the floor, circled around the popcorn bowl, all taking little mouthfuls while chatting away. Ellen, who had kept her interpretation of Lina's increasingly autistic behavior as similar to Pippi Longstocking's bold and unconventional but good-hearted overtures, was continuously intrigued by Lina's lack of awareness of social restrictions. She experienced Lina as free and fun-loving, someone who had the guts to live outside of the box. Hanging out at our place, without her parents around, Ellen wanted to have a taste of this freedom herself, and suddenly, without warning, smiled and took a whole handful of popcorn and chucked it across the room. We all, including Lina, looked at her with big eyes. This was something new. Elsa, excited by this unexpected role reversal, grabbed another handful and, with delight, threw it across the room. Within seconds, the room was snowing. Wholeheartedly, we all shared Lina's uninhibited, fearless, no-impulse-controlled state and before Valerie and I had any chance to think it over, most of the fruit-salad was sliding around the floor as well. It was a one-time thing, but it was the most genuine and heartfelt example of joining that I can think of. The Son-Rise people would have been delighted. The day ended with meat sauce and gluten-free pasta, just like in the old days when Anki and I alternated Wednesdays at our respective apartments, never serving anything but pasta and meat sauce and always ending our evenings with all four kids stuffed in the bathtub, Alfred doing his indoor slide trick. It wasn't particularly popular with the rest of the crew and involved him positioning himself on one of the short sides of the tub and sliding down on his bare rump, bumping into everyone and sending cascades of water out of the tub and onto the floor. But the pasta and meat sauce were everybody's favorite. For the past year or so, one of Lina's habits had been to eat her meals while sitting on top of the dinner table. This was clearly something Pippi Longstocking would do, and Ellen was not slow to follow suit. Soon, Elsa tried it out as well. Only Valerie and I remained on our chairs, smiling at Ellen's natural capacity to join and appreciate her old girlfriend's new and different world.

Sometimes, when Lina's unusual and intense behaviors elicited more decisive and firm responses in those around her, Lina responded with more clarity. Such was the case one evening before going to bed when she, without warning, whacked me in the face after biting me lightly in my arms and shoulders and simultaneously saying, "No biting." The powerful, sudden hit felt as if she'd broken my nose. Instinctively defending myself, I pushed Lina away from me onto the other mattress. She didn't like that, laughed half-heartedly, and then whimpered and came back to me. "Lina," I explained, "you can't hit. It hurts me and it's not okay. I love you very much but you absolutely can't hit." We were both quiet for a while. Then Lina spontaneously said, "I love you," and as if to make sure I would know it wasn't echolalia (her just repeating what I had said), she leaned toward me and put her soft cheek on mine. "I love you," she said again.

During the late spring, I went for Lina's first New York City IEP (Individualized Educational Plan) meeting. Sitting in the Board of Education's waiting room on 125th Street, waiting for the social worker to call us for Lina's first interview, I was struck by how different every kid was. Lina was the most active. She skipped around as usual, as if the place was her second home, approaching strangers to make little close-up studies of their faces, mothers and children alike, exploring their snacks, and spreading around that unlimited, unrestricted, open-hearted and heart-warming smile that makes most people melt and accept her little food thefts and boundary indiscretions.

When we met with Dr. Rubio, one of the Committee of Special Education's (CSE) child psychologists, Lina was in a particularly great mood—active and interested in everything Dr. Rubio said and stating yes or no and adding "Mama" to all of her requests. Five minutes into the interview, Lina had already managed to mark Dr. Rubio's sweater and pants with dark blackberry spots but he took it in stride. The interview ended with Dr. Rubio agreeing with the theory that Lina's challenges have very specific neurological roots, triggered by the MMR shot, subsequent Epstein-Barr virus, and the seizure and drooling episode that followed. There is an increasing volume of research confirming cerebral seizure susceptibility after measles, mumps, and rubella (MMR) vaccinations, possibly caused by concurrent viruses, which can damage the brain and cause pathology in not-yet mature immune systems and result in pervasive developmental disorder (PDD) and autism diagnoses. We might never know if the vaccine caused the autism in a legal sense, or whether it triggered some pre-existing vulnerability.

As always, aside from whatever new or old insight about Lina that could be gained through the numerous evaluations my daughter has undergone, one of the most important outcomes of any such meeting is always that we managed to come out of it in one piece. So it was this time, with the only slight side-tracking coming from the fact that Lina, right after the inter-view, threw chewing gum that landed smack in the middle of a big-breasted woman's cleavage. Luckily, the fellow parent, who was doing nothing but sitting innocently in the CSE waiting room gearing up for her own interview, responded with a broad, open-minded, and forgiving smile. I always want to hug such people for accepting my daughter as she is, and for not taking themselves so seriously that they can't see the humor in our crazy existence.

Within a couple of weeks, Lina had skipped through the CSE hallways with social workers, a psychologist, a psychiatrist, and a speech therapist to evaluate her functioning in all areas related to the issue of what school setting would be recommended. Lina continued her habit of confusing and intriguing evaluators with her happy, affectionate, and hyperactive presence. She was nothing like the other children, they said, but eventually, during the official IEP meeting that I attended without Lina, they recommended the most intensive setting for Lina that New York public school system could offer, which involved classes with six children and two adults, in specially designed classrooms to facilitate learning for kids with special needs. These special placements for children who cannot be integrated into the general public schools are administrated all around the city by what is referred to as district 75.

I went to visit and watched with skepticism as children a year older than Lina sat in a neat circle on the floor in the nice-looking but cluttered classroom, answering questions only when called upon, seeming to manage their days without bouncing balls, trampolines, or swings. *What does this place have to do with Lina?* I wondered to myself, but smiled and asked to see the cafeteria. It was lunchtime when I got there, loud and crowded with kids and teachers. The school representative pointed to a corner of the room where special-needs kids had their "educational meal." I left the school with a heavy heart. Lina would never survive in this setting. The teachers and assistants all seemed perfectly fine, but if I were to make an educated guess, Lina would have either escaped out onto the street or gotten herself suspended from the school within the first week. And even if they had let her stay, she needed so much more.

That idea of "more" came up in a conversation with a very approachable and lovely case manager at the Children's Resources Agency in Manhattan. I had explained to her the work we had done with Lina at home and how I thought Lina had too much integrity to be bribed by applied behavioral analysis (ABA), which was the most commonly utilized approach in the public school settings in New York City as well as in most other U.S. cities. ABA uses techniques for rewarding useful behaviors and reducing undesirable ones that I just didn't feel would work with Lina.

"Have you ever heard of the Rebecca School?" the case manager asked me.

It turned out to be a very important question. She went on to describe how this school was the only setting she knew of in Manhattan that was informed by a more relational approach like the one I hoped to find for Lina. After hanging up, I went to the Rebecca School's website and found out that it is a privately run school on the Lower East Side informed by the DIR model that was developed by psychiatrist Dr. Stanley Greenspan (now deceased but at that point an active force in the school). By now, I was a huge fan of Dr. Greenspan. But I had never heard about the school. I immediately called up their admissions office to schedule a visit. What I saw during my visit to numerous classrooms, watching how the kids related with such confidence and enthusiasm to genuinely warm and friendly teachers and teacher's assistants, was like winning a million dollars in the lottery, only much, much better. I went home, put my girls to bed, and sat down to write a letter to the admissions committee at Rebecca School. It was a long letter that involved descriptions of Lina as an "affectionate, fun-loving, and action-oriented" little girl who had come a long way compared to where she was at the onset of her difficulties. The letter ended as follows:

> *Hearing about your school, learning that you are guided by the DIR model and Greenspan, looking at your curriculum, reading about your work in dyads and small groups as well as your emphasis on social and emotional development as the foundation for all learning, made me overjoyed. For the first time in what feels like a long time, I saw a vision of a bridge between home and school.*

Soon, Lina and I were invited for a meeting with Liz, the admissions director, a tall, warm woman with red curly hair that suited her bubbly personality and the humorous gleam in her eyes. We also met with the clinical director, Dr. Gil Tippy, who, while not as outgoing as his colleague, revealed a more low-keyed intensity whenever broaching the subject of floor time and the DIR model. Dr. Tippy had brought a video camera for our meeting. He asked Lina and me to "have fun" while he recorded us. Lina did have "fun." I didn't. The room was full of unknown temptations. She already knew all about the clay that I had brought with me to demonstrate her budding ability for pretend play. Her putting a piece of the clay in her mouth was as close as we got to engaging with each other on tape. The cabinets up above the sink in the corner of the room were much more interesting. And there were some materials she was really interested in. Play-Doh, salty and with real wheat, was much better than clay to put in the mouth, and before anyone had a chance to stop her, half of the container was in her mouth. With a big grin, she proceeded to dump some bubble soap on the floor, ran across the room, jumped on the bouncing ball, ran back to the cabinets, was stopped this time by Dr. Tippy, and took off into the hallway. After that there was a mad rush in and out of all the other classrooms. My only comfort at that point was that Dr. Tippy couldn't possibly have caught it all on tape. She was moving too fast. "Well," said Dr. Tippy , a few minutes into the mad dashes in the hallway, including some jumping and screaming, "I think I've seen what I needed to see." With heavy heart, Lina and I exited the school. Lina didn't know that she probably had just ruined her chances to come to a school that was more interested in having a relationship with her than making her memorize the alphabet.

A few days later, I called the admissions director and asked her if it would be appropriate to submit a videotape of Lina at home to "complement your understanding of her."

"Sure," Liz agreed, and our new project was on its way.

The next couple of weeks were centered on catching Lina's most interactive, expressive, and peaceful moments on tape. It was fun. I recorded Lina and us at all different moments through the day. There was even an edited bathtub scene in the mix. A month later, Liz called me up when Lina and I were riding the elevator at the Jewish Community Center on the Upper West Side (one of Lina's favorite pastimes) to tell me that Lina had been accepted. My sense of euphoria was indescribable. There was a place for Lina in this world, a place that prioritized all the things that were so important to Lina at this time of her life. This place welcomed her in spite of her extreme intensity, in spite of the never-subsiding energy level that intimidated so many. Lina would have a place to belong to, outside of home. I felt so relieved and happy for her. There was no doubt in my mind that this was the right place for her. Tony, who also had come by for a tour of the school a couple of weeks after Lina's and my disastrous interview, felt equally happy to give our daughter this opportunity to expand her world. And while the school was not free, we hoped to impress upon the board of education that this was what Lina needed and get her schooling funded by them. We were only partially successful in this. The board of education paid for Lina's first year. Tony and I spent all of the next year going to meeting after meeting for hearings to try to explain to the board of education why Lina wouldn't have been successful in the placements we had been offered and had needed the alternative that Rebecca School provided. Eventually the judge ruled in our favor only to have the Department of Education attorney appeal his decision. The process seemed endless and was only recently resolved in our favor.

Lina started at Rebecca School during the summer of 2009. Many of the children there have IEPs (Individual Educational Plans) that involve twelve months of school rather than an extended summer break. Including vacations, that still doesn't add up to more than about ten months altogether. But it did allow Lina to start in the summer when it was a little less crowded and things were a little more relaxed than the rest of the year. Jill was Lina's new teacher. Her eyes sparkled with enthusiasm as she spoke of her classroom, the kids in it, and, almost immediately, about Lina. I stayed around, first together with Lina in the classroom and eventually in the parents' lounge, to be ready if Lina needed to check in with me. Lina wasn't actually spending much time in the classroom that first week. But she was fine, exploring the rest of the school and riding in the elevator to the other floors, accompanied by various teachers and assistants. She would press the elevator buttons and have little one-on-one conversations with whoever was following along.

One of the assistants was Darla. She had long, dark hair and intense brown eyes, dressed in hip little outfits, and had a big, uninhibited smile that caught Lina's heart from her first week of school. Darla and Lina became an entity. When I delivered Lina on my bike (I had kept her as my backseat co-pilot throughout the years even as she got taller and older; she still loved riding in the seat behind me, occasionally hugging me, talking about the various foods she would love to eat when we got to wherever we were going), Darla was the one waiting outside the school building every morning. She would come up to us with her big, contagious smile and even when Lina had trouble separating from me, it was Darla's shoulders she preferred to cry on. When Lina ran around the play-yard up on the school's roof, Darla was the one chasing her. When both Tony and I had to go to the next IEP meeting, Darla was the one hanging out with our girl in the sensory gym at Rebecca School where Lina could swing, climb, hide in little tunnels, and roll around the thick mats covering the floor. During the fall semester, Darla was reassigned to another classroom, working with older children. Angry and brokenhearted, Lina wouldn't speak to Darla in the hallways around the school for the first three months. Then, in the spring of 2010, Darla came back to Jill's classroom, and Lina was back in her friend's arms. Darla had come into Lina's life just as Valerie left us and our shared New York existence for a new life in Connecticut with her boyfriend. Luckily, our old babysitter and family friend, Therese, came back into our lives during that time, spending some time with us each week and helping Lina and Elsa understand that in the face of so many personal losses, some friends and babysitters reappear and new friends come along.

At Rebecca School, Lina also met a friend close to her own age. Fedi was in the same class as Lina though one year older. She took Lina under her wing from Lina's first day of school. At the beginning, before Fedi learned the hard way that Lina can only be enticed, never forced, to do anything, Fedi would lie flat on the classroom floor, wailing, "LINA, I WANT LINA!" She would lie there, inconsolable, yearning for her new friend whenever Lina was out touring the school, riding around in the elevator. Fedi felt so intensely betrayed by Lina's regular elevator expeditions that she started to go with her. The two of them took their rides together, visiting various classrooms, popping other children's balloons and tasting their snacks whenever possible, and making their mark on every floor. Lina, like Fedi, made friends with teachers and assistants on every floor. Soon, the odd couple, Lina with her unruly, blond-reddish curls and lean, muscular physique, and Fedi, with her black braids, brown skin, and strong, robust body, acted like two rock stars touring the country, hand-slapping and high-fiving their way through the corridors.

CHAPTER SEVEN

Spiritual Healing

Lina and I were wandering around Central Park. It was winter and very few people had found their way to what had become a second home for Lina and me. Lina looked at the lake next to the wooded area north of the boat-house where our wanderings always seemed to end up. I looked at her looking and commented, "Cold ice."

"Frozen," Lina responded, spontaneously and without any prompting, showing me her newly regained ability to make connections, generalize, and share her experiences verbally.

Later that day, as we were back home, Lina came up to me. Looking into my eyes and with a poise and awareness that most people have trouble attaining even in adulthood, she said:

"Everything is gonna be okay."

Before Lina was born, during pregnancy, my good friend Roseanne, who at the time was a candidate at the psychoanalytic institute where I had also studied, told me about a premonition she'd had about my unborn child. She thought it was a boy, which even now is what most people who meet Lina assume. While Lina is a beautiful child, she looks like a boy and talks like a boy. Roseanne, who died of cancer a few months after this conversation, laughingly told me that this child would be a very active child.

"I can imagine that," I said.

"No, no," Roseanne, said, "No, Helena, I don't think you can imagine. . . . This child is gonna be something else. I see him running around like crazy, everyone chasing him. Oh, boy, Helena, you got your work cut out for you."

"Oh yeah?"

"Mmm," Roseanne smiled, "a little wild one, wonderful, warm, *very* active."

Coming from a regimented Christian upbringing that seemed to focus more on sins and guilt and shortcomings than on joy, peace, and infinity, I had trouble practicing and defining my own faith. But when my life became more and more defined by frightening and exhausting changes in Lina, turning our whole family's life around, I felt that I had no choice. I had to find something beyond my own ability. Eventually, I realized, it wasn't beyond my ability.

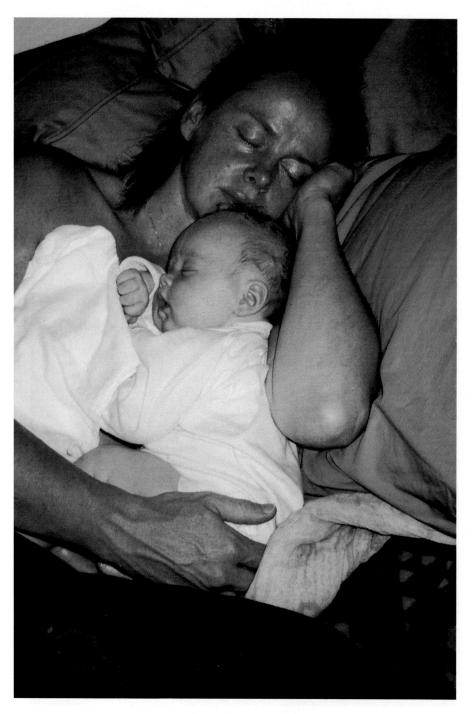

Baby Lina and me sleeping

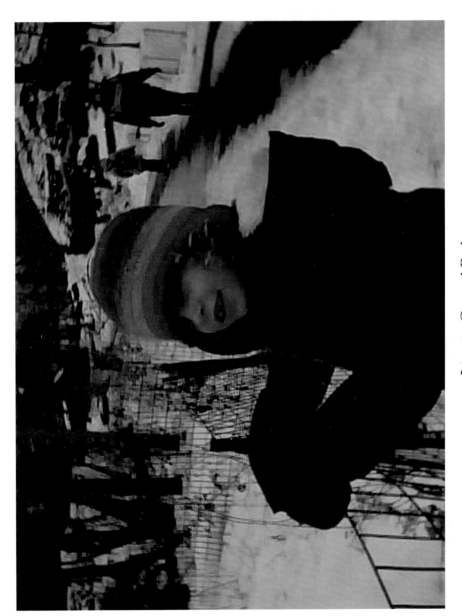

Lina in Central Park

Elsa and Lina

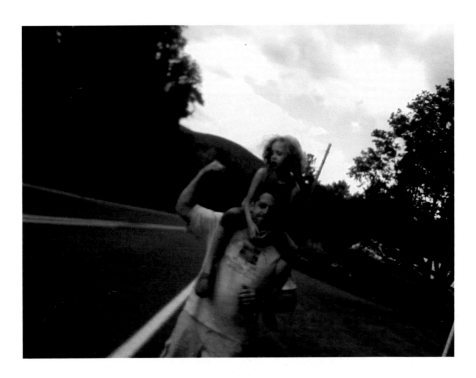

Lina and Tony

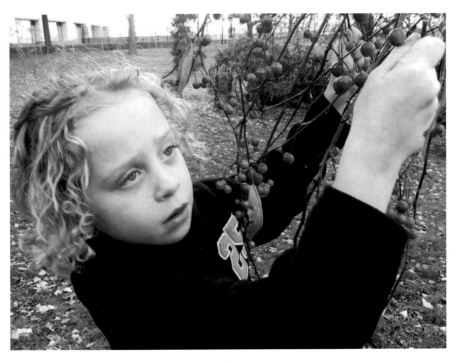

Lina

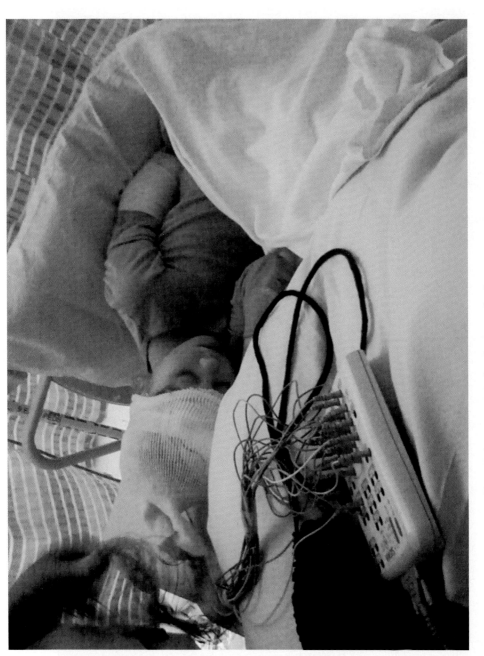

Lina sleeping in the hospital after more seizures

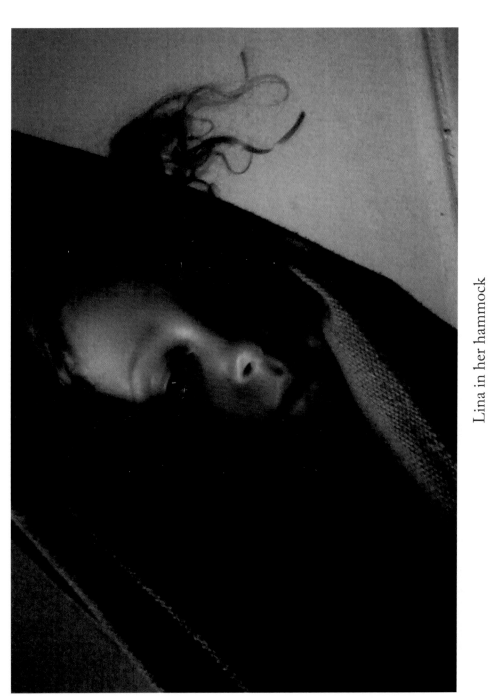

Lina in her hammock

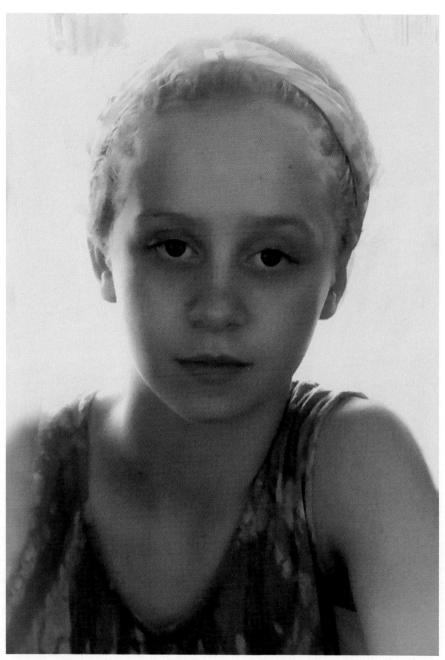

Lina's 12th birthday

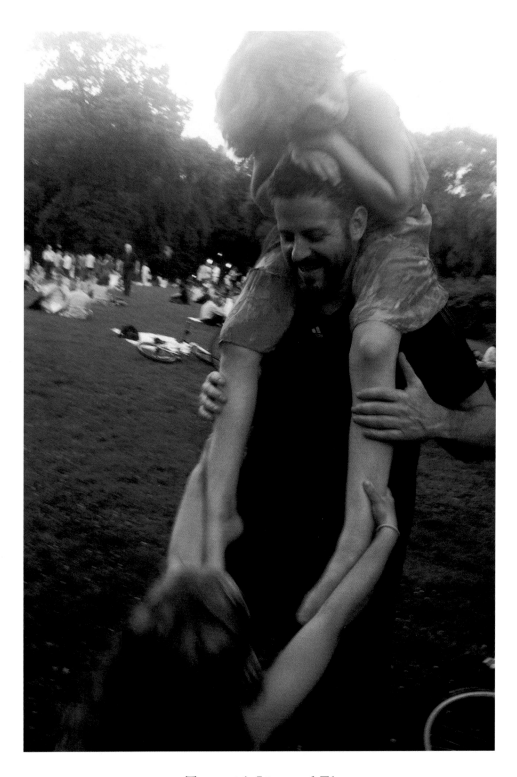

Tony with Lina and Elsa

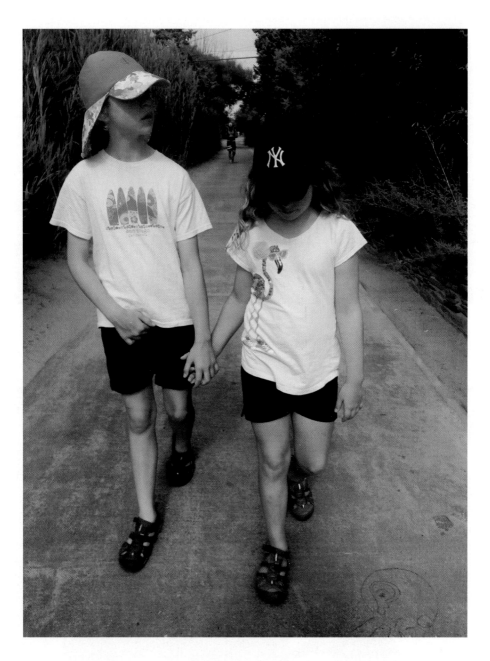

Lina and Elsa

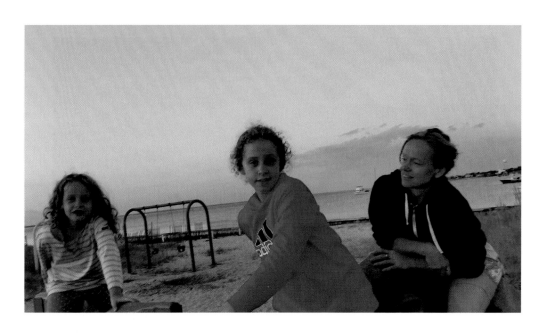

Lina and Elsa and me

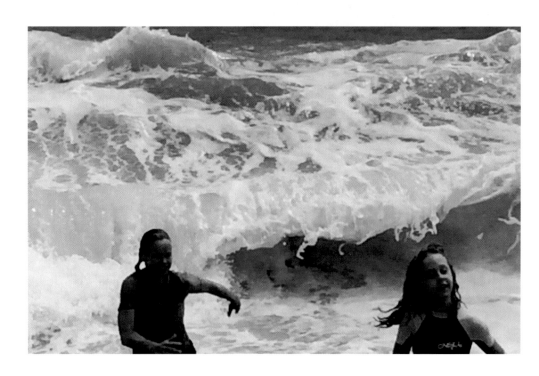

Running from a giant wave with Lina

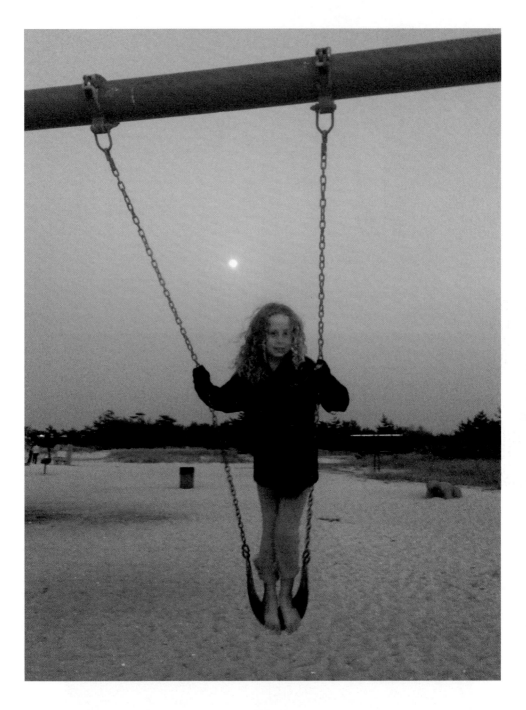

Lina

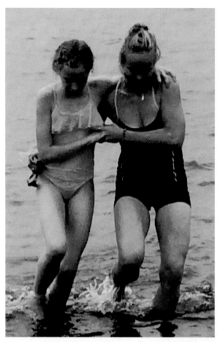

Lina and me in calm
waters

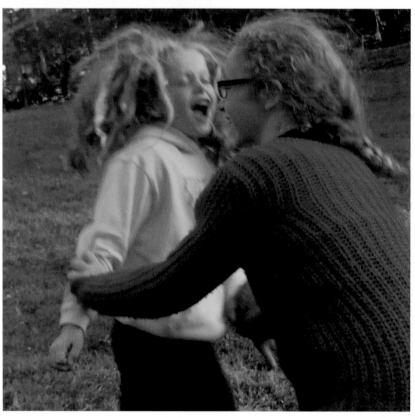

Elsa and Lina celebrating Native American Day
(formerly known as Columbus Day)

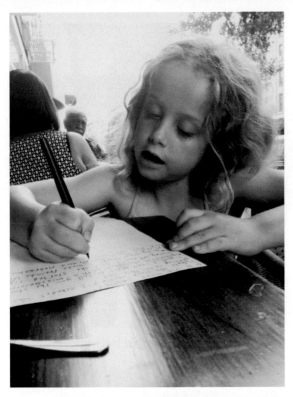

Elsa

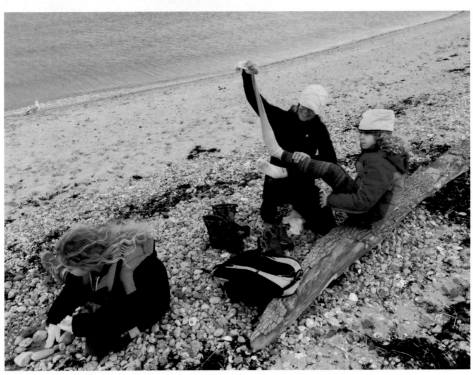

After Lina's spontaneous Winter swim

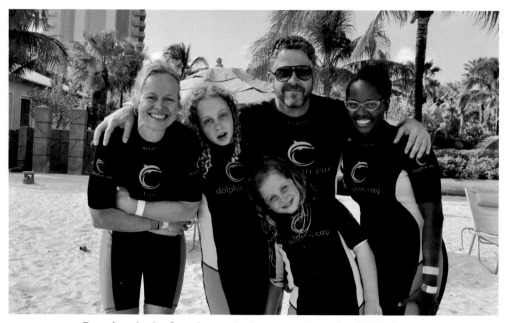

Lina's whole family, including our wonderful babysitter
Roshelle, on vacation

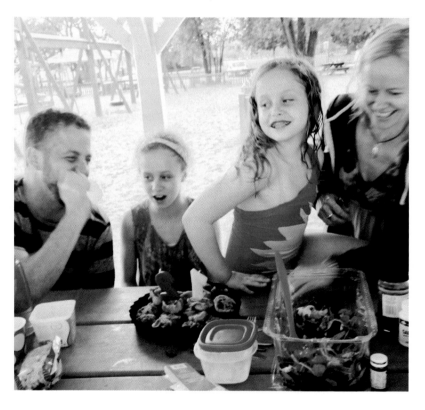

Lina's 12th birthday

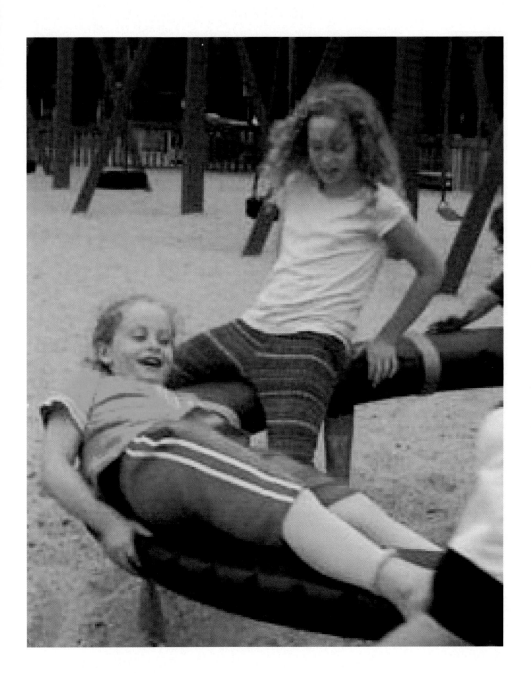

Elsa and Lina

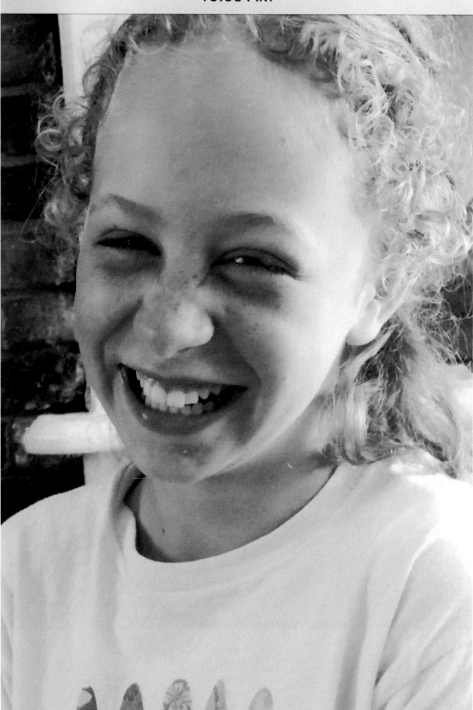

During Lina's sixth and seventh years, I felt that Lina was most receptive when I honored our spiritual connection. It is not hard to do with a child like Lina. She is so much more readily communicative on that level than when verbal responses and words are expected or even demanded. Alone at home on dark winter nights, I pray, sing, and talk to Lina, sometimes guided by an approach developed by the Hawaiian shaman Serge Kahili King called the "Dynamind Technique" (see *Healing for the Millions—The Amazing Dynamind Technique,* by Serge Kahili King, 2004). Using this method, one focuses on a concrete issue and then states the wish for it to heal or transform in the context of a very simple ritual that involves gestures and a breathing technique. Daily, I stated Lina's difficulties finding her words and asked the spiritual world to help her find them. I asked for the chance to get to know her better, to have a dialogue, and for Lina to have a chance to develop her connection with her sister and to be able to play with her. Furthermore, I asked for retrospective healing for Lina from the time when she was about three and a half—the time of the first signs of her difficulties.

Often, I also verbalized these prayers at bedtime, together with Lina and Elsa, before singing them to sleep. They would both listen carefully, and then Elsa would join in with some of her own prayers, often involving a whole row of "thank you Gods" and lists of who she loves (Mama and Papa and sometimes Lina, when she doesn't scream, as well as a few others currently on her mind) and hopes that Lina would fall asleep soon and not scream and jump around. Occasionally, Lina would add "thank you" as well, but most of the time she would listen for a while and then start to self-talk about her favorite subject, food.

One night, as I was singing and praying for Lina, alone in my office after the girls had fallen to sleep, I heard myself singing the word *ashia*, over and over. Afterward, I looked up the meaning of the word and found that its Arabic meaning is *life* and *hope*. When I picked up Lina the next day at school, one of the teacher's assistants, Tamar, mentioned that both she and Lina's teacher Jill and another teacher's assistant in a different classroom had been struck by how much Lina had been talking today. On the way home, Lina answered my question about what she had for lunch.

"Sprouts," she said.

"Yes, I remember packing that . . . what did you just say?"

Lina who almost never answered questions, had just told me what had been in her lunch! Later that day, Lina and I were standing outside Elsa's friend Aubrey's house. The door to their lobby was locked and we were waiting for Maria, Aubrey's babysitter, to buzz us in. Impatiently, Lina turned to me and said, "We need the keys!"

That night, I expressed my gratitude for Lina's verbal and conceptual breakthrough and continued to ask for Lina to "come back to us," visualizing her brain neurons making increasingly efficient connections and for the neuro pathways between various parts of her brain to communicate better with each other. I asked for Lina to regain her ability to play and talk about her feelings and thoughts when she was ready and for healing for me from that time when I was in a dark, shut down place myself. As I was singing, tears and deep sadness surfaced and the word *ari* came to me over and over in the song. Looking it up afterward, I saw that *ari*, in the Maori language, means "visible, clear." Looking further, I saw that *ari* is also a name with Scandinavian origin, and means *lion*. Lina was born on July 30. She is a lion.

During this time, Lina's expressiveness became more consistent, and she also revealed a more expressive awareness of others around her. One evening as Lina and Elsa and I were having dinner, Elsa was reminiscing about their friends in Rhode Island, Kevin, Alicia, Burke, and Eric (Lauren and Michael's children). I said we'll see them again one day. Lina joined in the conversation and said, "We will all have grapes together!"

Her optimism about maintaining old friendships in spite of the distance between us made me particularly happy since she had lost so many people close to her, including Valerie. And yet, she welcomed new and old people in her life. Sean, a young man in his mid-twenties, joined us in 2009 and is still with us. Every time Sean comes into my apartment to work with Lina in the playroom or be with Elsa while I'm with Lina, with his sweet, good-natured here-I-am-willing-and-able-smile, I am thankful for the very special blessing of Sean. He is no less than an angel. When my girlfriends with kids want to have him, too, I tell them he is not for rent.

Another day, Lina, Elsa, Sean, and I entered a snow-covered park, realizing that we should have brought our sled. We were discussing whether I should run back to the apartment and get it when Lina, in that same community spirit as when she'd contemplated sharing grapes, ran up the hill, smiling at us and shouting, "It will be fun!"

Back home Lina wanted me to read one of her favorite books, *Waves in the Bathtub*. Delighted that she asked, I dropped what I was doing and came into the room to join her. With that same large communal spirit, she smiled and said, "Welcome!"

As I dropped Lina off at school one day, Elisabeth, the woman who pulled Lina out of the classroom at Rebecca School on an almost daily basis for floor time, wanted to talk to me. Lina and Elisabeth had a deep connection, and Elisabeth, who makes her own decision about which child to work with, took an interest in Lina. Every time I saw this woman in the hallways of the school or with Lina in the sensory gym, I felt so grateful. We had an understanding: there is more to life than what's on the surface. Lina communicates on different levels. We listen to every level, not just the verbal. When Elisabeth pulled me into an empty room outside Lina's classroom, she said, "I want to tell you something."

I looked at Elisabeth and saw that whatever it was that she had to tell me, it was personally meaningful to her.

"Before the Christmas break, Lina kept telling me something. She said, 'Death.' She would pull my arm now and then and just say this word to me, 'death!' I didn't understand so I just said, 'Okay, Lina, death, okay,' and then we would just go on doing what we were doing. I didn't think more about it then, but during the Christmas break, my father died. So now I understand that she was trying to tell me that. And I thought I wanted to tell you this."

Elisabeth's story, and much of Lina's communication directly to me, reminded me of how important it was to listen to Lina, really listen and give space for her to communicate in whatever way comes most easily to her.

It's easy to get sidetracked, to lose one's center, to become disintegrated and distracted like Lina. And it is so easy to try to cover up one's unease by trying to dominate the situation instead of remaining sensitive to Lina's experience. But she senses discomfort, imbalance, frustration, anger, and insecurity in others much more acutely than most of us. The more comfortable I am with myself, the more centered and peaceful, the better she responds. She might test it for a while. She might challenge it to see if it's real, but soon, if my peace and comfort stand the test of her screams and throwing things across the room or grabbing something from the refrigerator and running around the apartment with it, she settles down. Often, silence is the best communicator. Wordless communication from a place of peace and stillness, with slow, sincere movements, helps her come back to herself and reconnect with her own center. One day we were sitting under a tree that had tiny little red apples growing from its branches. In my mind, I asked myself, "Should I ask Lina what color the little apples are?" "Red!" Lina responded, before I had a chance to finish the thought. I called Tony to give him yet another example of how Lina reads minds. "Send her to Harvard," he teased me as he often did whenever I talked about Lina's latest achievement. But the next day Tony called me. He had picked up Lina from school. He had not had time to eat lunch and was starving. As soon as Lina saw him, and before he had even had a chance to say hello to his little daughter, she looked straight at him and said, "You are hungry."

For the first time since Lina was born, I traveled alone, for more than one night, without the girls. My close friend Gabriella, who lives in Spain, was visiting her younger brothers in Los Angeles for two months and I decided to go and see her. Gabriella is a shaman. All through her life, she has searched for what's beyond our physical reality. She has studied under Hawaiian Huna shamans, Siberian shamans, and even traveled to Peru to be initiated by the Queros' shamans. Through stones, cards, maracas, and incense, motivated by her own strong wish to be helpful, to be who she feels she is meant to be, she takes journeys through people's past, present, and future. She is connected with what the eye cannot see and willing to let go of conscious thoughts and awareness during her rituals, to see more clearly what's beyond consciousness and the material world.

I left on a Monday after dropping Lina off at school and came back two days later. A short trip, and yet I was only barely able to follow through with it. The last time I had been away from the girls, when Lina and Elsa had gone with Tony to Woodstock over the weekend, Lina was furious at me when they came back and sang loudly and angrily, "I'VE BEEN WAITING A LOOONG TIME!" Then she punched me with her clenched fist and repeated, "I'VE BEEN WAITING A LONG TIME!!" It took her an hour, a lot of high-pitched screaming and crying, and two serious bite marks, one of which punctured the skin on my forearm, the other on my shoulder, to calm down before her face opened into a heart-warming smile and she wrapped her little strong arms around my neck. So I definitely planned to have a long-sleeved shirt on at my return from L.A. But this time was different. Lina didn't know it, but one reason for the trip, apart from just being with my very dear friend, was that she and I would spend some time doing shamanic journeying together. Without going into the details of this very personal healing experience, I came back feeling like I had been away on a two-month vacation rather than just two days. Lina knew. Jill, her teacher, reported to me that when I was away, Lina had spontaneously talked about my trip, saying that, "Mama is going to get good."

More intensively than anyone else in my life, Lina is my teacher. She is my opportunity and ongoing reminder to become a little more free. A little less trapped. A little less of a victim of my circumstances as well as of my own expectations. With Lina, having expectations of what any given day is going to be like is not useful. Openness and acceptance make it much more possible to get through the day sane. Lina has not only helped me to relate less rigidly to who and how she should be but to who I should be and what kind of life I should have as well. At the same time, acceptance, somehow, has to encapsulate all of us: Elsa, Tony, Sean, Lina's teachers, and anyone else involved in our lives. It's not just a matter of accepting Lina's every behavior. We are interconnected. Everyone in the family needs to have the right to feel what they feel, to say no, to cry, to get mad. Without that, it's not going to work. Continually, Lina helps expand my acceptance of myself. As Lina is developing further, she has less and less difficulty accepting when I say no. As long as I do it without ambivalence, clearly and firmly, preferably with a slightly elevated tone of voice, she often seems to relax into it. I have realized that one of the most important lessons in my relationship with Lina is to respect my own boundaries, my own limitations, my own "NO!"

Gabriella advised me to look up the Daimoko, a Buddhist chant that Nichiren Buddhists chant as their primary practice. This chant—Nam-Myoho-Renge-Kyo—represents a kind of compressed version of the most essential teachings in the Lotus Sutra. It was the Buddhist Nichiren, born in Japan in 1222, who devoted himself to teaching the "Wonderful Law of the Lotus Flower Sutra" or Nam-Myoho-Renge-Kyo, to everyone, regardless of educational background and intellectual ability. Nichiren believed that simply chanting the Daimoko made it possible for anyone with a sincere faith to find enlightenment. Nichiren

Buddhism is different from many other forms of Buddhist philosophy in that it does not require that we renounce our desire. In *The Buddha in Your Mirror* (2001, p. 40) by Woody Hochswender, Greg Martin, and Ted Morino, the authors describe how "Nichiren stated that the source of all desire is life itself; as long as life continues, we instinctively want to live, to cherish love, to seek profit. . . . Since desire arises from the innermost core of life, it is virtually indestructible. Even the thirst for enlightenment is a kind of desire."

Here was a chant and a Buddhist philosophy that didn't force me to stop praying for Lina's full recovery from every aspect of autism that brought her further away from us. I did not have to transform my desire for her to play and communicate and be calm and comfortable and connected with everyone around her into something "higher." I could just chant away. In my daily practice were reminders of the Shoten Zenjin—protective forces of nature, occurrences that are not humanly possible. Here was room, not just for gratitude and interconnectedness with all life, but also for my personal wishes, in the present as well as in the future. I felt relieved. Here was the bridge between Shamanism and Buddhism that I'd been looking for. In this practice was room for me and my girls, happiness and peace, friends and lovers. It became the daily practice that is helping me become who I feel I am supposed to be. And I believe, through my prayers and Gabriella's prayers and through everyone who helps me pray and work for Lina's full return from her isolated rooms of autism, this is one of the essential aspects of what will bring her back.

There is an inherent conflict in asking for someone to become who they are not. I love the way Lina is in this moment in the same way that I love who she has been in every single moment of her life. She is the most authentic, intuitive, magical human being I have ever met. But she lost many of the very essential functions that connect one human being to another in life as it is on this earth. She lost the ability to play and imagine, the comprehension of what is going on around her, the ability to make herself understood and to express things that are important to her, the ability to develop close friendships, the capacity to crack a joke. . . . and I know she is funny. But so many of the jokes are frozen inside of her. So much of her sadness can never quite be expressed and understood. So much of how she sees her world is lost to everyone around her. So absolutely, I want her back. Back to a time when she was running around the apartment feeding her doll and pretending that she was a master chef, feeding everyone around her, including me and Elsa, the most imaginative meals. So the chanting continues.

One Saturday morning, as Lina and Elsa and I were hanging out in the playroom, Lina got out of her hammock, climbed up in the window to fetch a little "troll-doll-girl" with long green hair and tail, brought it with her into the hammock, studied her face and hair, and smiled affectionately. I grabbed for the camera and got three amazing pictures of something that hadn't happened since Lina was three and a half years old. As if I didn't have enough to celebrate that day, an hour later, Lina went into the playroom, fetched a Pippi Longstocking puzzle, threw the pieces out of the frame onto the floor, and, on her own initiative, started putting the puzzle together again. A startled Elsa came and offered to help her. But Lina ended up helping Elsa. I just stared at my daughters, sitting there on the soft mat in the middle of the playroom, putting a puzzle together, the oldest modeling for the youngest. At three-and-a-half, Lina had been a master at puzzles. A friend of Tony's, a father himself, had seen Lina playing with puzzles in the living room and had commented that Lina seemed to be an especially gifted child. And here she was, right in front of me, doing something she hadn't been able to do for almost five years. I was flying for the rest of that day.

For me, chanting, meditation, and yoga, ongoing connecting with my own center, has become the most powerful medicine. I have found that finding resources beyond the physical world, beyond my own mind—inside, deep down, where past and future, thoughts and feelings don't rule—is, after years of searching on the outside for an answer that benefits Lina, the most important path to finding her. Of course, dietary issues, biomedical treatment, choices of school, and home therapy are extremely important. But not as important as what is happening on the inside. Lina already knows this. She has always remembered the character of Leelanau, a little girl who lives with her parents in a Native American village and who escapes to the forest. The trees and the peace in the forest are a very spiritual place for her, where she hangs out with the animals of the forest as well as with light, sparkling fairies called *puukwodjinees*. There, Leelanau is completely herself, free from the expectations of her parents, free from having to live according to the values, traditions, and customs of the culture she grew up with. Here, in the spacious, magical forest, she can connect with her own power, something inside of her that's intact and infinite. Her parents are afraid that they will lose Leelanau to the forest and the spiritual reality that she encountered there and want to arrange her marriage as a way of ensuring her ongoing presence in the village. Leelanau, longing for the freedom and spiritual life in the magical world of the forest where she is connected with everything and everyone around her as well as with the part of herself that will always be, runs away from home and never comes back.

Lina loved this book. Lately, I have been looking around for it. It's been lost for years, but the message wasn't lost on Lina. She understands Leelanau's longing to be who she is rather than living up to cultural and parental expectations of who she should be and what she should and should not do. Sometimes Lina will say, "Let's go to the spirit world." And I don't tell her not to go. I don't want to try to prevent her from going and risk losing her altogether, like Leelanau's parents did. I would rather she feel that being connected in the spiritual world helps her to put up with the ignorance and fearfulness and attachment in the material world. I would rather that now and then, both of us could travel to the spiritual world together. And I would rather she feel that her spiritual needs were respected and supported.

I felt so happy the day when Lina, on our way to school one cold, gray March morning, listened to me singing a Swedish spiritual goodnight song about being protected in God's hands, smiled, and said in a low voice, "Mama is going to the spirit world."

"Yes, my dear," I responded and smiled back, "we go there together, you and I."

Lina looked at me for a long time, clearly taking this in. When not with my children and not working, I had begun to do daily meditations, going into my bedroom and lying down on the bed with curtains pulled, thanking Lina and Elsa and the people close to me, including myself, for being who they are and for being in my life. It helped me stay present with myself and Lina and Elsa and others in my life. And it shifted the focus from feelings of burnout and fear of not being able to meet the challenges in my life the way I wanted to and the way that Lina and Elsa needed me to, to a sense of being lucky and whole.

Lina knows when I'm connected to myself and to her and when I'm distracted, anxious, and absentminded. One day we were walking by the Hudson River. Lina was picking beach plums. It was so peaceful. I turned to Lina and without thinking, out of the blue, I told her, "Lina, you don't have to choose. You can love both mama and papa. We both love you so much." She looked at me for a long time, like she always does before saying something that comes straight from her heart, as if to make sure I'm really taking it in:

"Sometimes we live in the same place."

At first, I thought she was referring to the idea of Tony and I living in different places and Lina sometimes being at Tony's place, but I think more that she may have been talking about how she and I understand each other. The idea of Lina not having to choose between being close to me or Tony had touched my daughter. Later that night, Lina and I bounced together on a large exercise ball to some music as we always do before bedtime. I noticed that the necklace my friend Gabriella had given me after her recent trip to Peru was a little sharp against Lina's chest when I held her close to me on the bouncing ball. So I took it off, putting it on the couch next to us. Lina took it and put it back around my neck. I turned it around so that the sharp stone was on my back. Lina moved it back to the front in between us, and with knowing, deliberate hand movements, she carefully arranged it on my chest before leaning in toward me, pressing against it.

My friend Gabriella described seeing me and Lina and Elsa right at the center of a tornado, in the eye of the tornado where everything is still. Stillness is sometimes the only thing that helps. Eckhart Tolle, in *Stillness Speaks* (2003, p. 77), writes:

> *We depend on nature not only for our physical survival. We also need nature to show us the way home, the way out of the prison of our own minds. We got lost in doing, thinking, remembering, anticipating—lost in a maze of complexity and a world of problems.*
> *We have forgotten what rocks, plants, and animals still know. We have forgotten how to be—to be still, to be ourselves, to be where life is: Here and Now.*

To Elsa's wonderful and very intelligent psychotherapist, in one of my updates before Elsa's appointment, I wrote:

> *There are ongoing challenges with Lina and this morning, Elsa was very explicitly upset about Lina's screaming, covering her ears with her hands, looking miserable and pissed off, talking about how she doesn't like the screaming. Lina, as is customary [during this phase], threw milk all over the kitchen, and her cereal started flying around soon after the milk. Lina was confused about the milk and cereal and there was also something else she wanted to say to Elsa but couldn't make herself understood. . . . I'm trying to just concentrate on one moment, one situation at the time. When I do well, and am calm and focused, it gives Elsa a chance to express her feelings, be more needy, etc. I've been spending time relating to myself as a daughter, not so much the daughter to my*

mother but in a broader sense, imagining Mother Earth, a
cosmic mother, the ground, trees, wind, water. . . . You may
think this sounds crazy but this is really helping me. It's an
extreme challenge we're in—all of us—and there isn't much
to be found in the physical environment so it makes sense
to me to find it beyond tangible reality. To me, this kind
of meditation makes me feel connected to something much
bigger than my own resources, and that, as I see it, is the only
way of living the day to day as it is at this point.

One Saturday morning after picking up Lina at Tony's place after having my weekly night without the kids, Lina and I were walking home. Sean had taken Elsa to the park. I had taken Lina to an empty playground in Central Park, and pushed her on a tire swing, with her smiling at me the whole time. On the way home I stopped for a moment and realized how lucky I was to have this unique connection with my almost eight-year-old daughter. Lina looked back at me and said, "Let's go home." I looked at my little girl, reaching up to my chest now, tall and slim and so beautiful and loving, and said: "I'm so glad that you're here with me. What would I do without you?" We got home and, unlike the way Lina usually hurries to throw her shoes and socks and jacket off in the corner by the door and run over to the refrigerator in her search for something to eat, she calmly walked over to me and wrapped her arms around me, just stood there quietly, opening up a kind of sacred space and awareness between us that is so rare in many people's relationships where words replace and fill up and distract from so much of that needed space. I again just felt so lucky.

Another such magic moment happened when Lina and I were on the bus, on our way back home from school. A very tall, older man who sat next to us sang a song in a different language. I had never heard it but it filled the bus with a peaceful feeling. I smiled. The old man had a beautiful voice and his face was open and relaxed. He smiled back and said, "I have to sing. Otherwise I'll go crazy, these times; it's so hard to find work. But singing helps me."

"Singing heals everything," I said.

We all sat quiet for a moment. Then Lina started singing a similar melody with words that sounded like the same language as what the man had just sung.

"Does she go to church?" the man asked me.

"No, her church is inside of her."

"She is singing a song from church," the man told me, looking confused at first, then smiled and started singing again.

I turned to Lina who turned to me, leaned forward, and stroked my cheek as if to say, "It's okay, Mama, you don't have to understand everything about me."

Lina and I went to the playground by the Hudson River late one beautiful, sunny August day. Walking next to her, slowly approaching the playground, felt wonderful. Tony and I had just had some tension about the fact that both of our schedules didn't seem to offer much time for anything other than work and being with the girls. But the late August sun, and Lina's hand in mine, melted my tension away. But, by the time we got to the playground, Lina, who is hypersensitive to conflict and tension between people around her, was ready to process *her* experience. She screamed on the swing. Ran away without her shoes. She went into the standing-water puddles in the middle of the playground with her clothes still on. She picked up chewing gum from the ground and refused to spit it out.

I had a fresh bite-mark from Lina between my neck and shoulder that hadn't healed yet. It was still painful a few days after the fact but had healed up enough for me to decide not to go to the hospital to have it checked out. It was much deeper than any other bite that I had gotten from Lina. Her biting, during the summer of 2010, had slowly made its reappearance. The closer she was with someone, the more likely she was to bite. Both Valerie and Sean learned this the hard way. Tony knows, too. Only Elsa is exempted from this list. Lina doesn't ever bite Elsa. She has pushed her and slapped her and even kicked lightly, but she will not bite her little sister. Half an hour into this playground time, Lina wanted to be picked up for comfort. But she was still frustrated and tense and bit right into the still open sore next to my neck and then whacked me in my face. Something very strong welled up inside of me. The pain was unbearable.

My mind went off. How can it be that I have a child that hurts me like an attacking animal? I felt hatred. I wanted to hit her back, bite her, or throw her down on the ground. Instead, I pushed her to the ground and, with fear and rage in my face and voice, told her that if she ever did that again I would fight back, I would bite her or hit her because I simply couldn't live with this anymore. As I spoke those words, I felt that in that moment, I could carry out my threat. The gap between saying it, warning her, and actually doing felt very small. It terrified both of us. Eventually we calmed down and sat down on the lawn next to the playground, looking out on the river. We sat there quietly for what felt like a long time and then slowly made our walk back home. The rest of our afternoon was calm and connected. At some point, in the kitchen, as

I was quietly singing "Amazing Grace," Lina looked at me, smiled with that knowing look in her eyes, leaned forward, and said: "Sorry, sorry." She kept smiling and then again said, "Sorry, sorry."

"I'm sorry, too, baby, I know you didn't mean it. And I didn't mean what I said either. I will get mad at you and sometimes I will be furious at you, but I would never hit you back, no matter what you do. I love you very much."

The following day was Sunday, and I had the afternoon to myself. Lina was back at the same playground with Elissa, one of our babysitters. Knowing how Lina's visual memory works, I was aware that the best way for me to deal with what happened the day before would be to deal with it now. So I hopped on the bike back to the place of the disaster. Predictably, as soon as Lina saw me, she started yelling and saying, "No, no!" She wanted me to leave. Then she wanted me to stay. Then she wanted me to pick her up. I put her on my shoulders this time and took a deep breath. At first, the rhythmical movement of me swaying from side to side calmed her. Then, the visual memory of yesterday took over and she bit me, hard, on the top of my head. This time I was prepared. I knew what I was there to do. I gently but firmly pushed her head in the direction of the biting to lessen the impact and calmly but firmly said, "No, Lina, it's not okay to bite." Eventually, she let go. I lifted her down. She looked at me and said, "It is tough!" I hugged her and responded, "I know, my angel. Thank you for telling me. I know it is tough. I'm sorry I got so mad at you yesterday. I love you, Lina, and I'll see you later." Back home, I picked up *The Power of Now—A Guide to Spiritual Enlightenment*, by Eckhart Tolle, and read:

So whenever your relationship is not working, whenever it brings out the "madness" in you and your partner, be glad. What was unconscious is being brought up to the light. It is an opportunity for salvation. Every moment, hold the knowing of that moment, particularly of your inner state. If there is anger, know that there is anger . . . an inner child demanding love and attention, or emotional pain of any kind—whatever it is, know the reality of that moment and hold the knowing. The relationship then becomes your sadhana, your spiritual practice (p. 158).

I think we all have those very special teachers in our lives. A lover, a husband or wife, a child, a close friend, an employer, a colleague. Lina is my greatest *sadhana*. It's not just me. She teaches everyone she cares about. But as her mother, I get special lessons. Tolle (1997, p. 159) continues:

But if you accept that the relationship is here to make you conscious instead of happy, then the relationship will offer you salvation, and you will be aligning yourself with the higher consciousness that wants to be born into this world.

That night, Elsa stayed at Tony's house and Lina and I had the evening together, just the two of us. At bedtime I listened to her breathing and felt so lucky, lying there quietly next to her. Lina responded to my wordless expression of gratitude by snuggling closer to me.

CHAPTER EIGHT

A Father's Love

In the early spring of 2010, Tony co-wrote a book with Ken Siri, parent of Alex, a student at Rebecca School, called *Cutting-Edge Therapies for Autism*, that compiles the latest advances in treatment. During this project, Tony, who would come to my apartment in the mornings as he was bringing one of the girls to school, began dropping enthusiastic statements about the various treatments represented in the book. My head was spinning. Every day, Tony presented a new theory, dismissing the one he had glowed over the previous morning. One of the chapters in his book was written by Dr. Michael

Goldberg, on "Neuroimmune Dysfunction and the Rationale and Use of Antiviral Therapy."

Goldberg describes how children with diagnoses of autism often have hyperactive and dysfunctional immune systems that make them susceptible to secondary infection with chronic viruses that eventually attack the brain. In treating children with hyperactive immune systems, or autoimmune disorders, Dr. Goldberg begins with what he calls "reversing the negatives." Negatives are all the foods that make these children's immune systems overreact. In other words, any food that boosts one's immune system, such as fruit rich in vitamin C, is a negative for a child with a hyperactive immune system. Subsequently, Dr. Goldberg recommends eliminating foods that trigger reactions or act as stimulants to the immune systems of children with autism spectrum disorder (ASD). Goldberg talks about the very common appearance of an "immune-stressed" state in children diagnosed with ASD, where simple autoimmune disorders such as eczema, congestion, or allergies develop into more severely dysfunctional neuroimmune systems causing symptoms common in children with autism. Goldberg describes how ASD children's hyperreactive immune systems eventually can lead to a "neuroimmune shutdown." Over time, Dr. Goldberg's thoughts on the relationship between autism spectrum disorders, the immune system, and neuroimmune dysfunction seemed particularly relevant to Lina. Dietary issues are always at the forefront for us and for many families with a child with autism. Gastrointestinal troubles are a common thread. Lina had been on a gluten-free, casein-free, sugar-free diet for most of the time since the onset of her difficulties. After some intermittent attempts to reintroduce milk and bread and a little bit of sugar into her diet, we have concluded that Lina seems better off staying off milk, bread, and sugar.

The diet Goldberg proposed, called "the antiviral diet," seemed worth trying. According to Goldberg, not only dairy products and sugar were disqualified as appropriate for Lina, but also all sorts of whole grains and rice, nuts, and most fruits such as berries and citrus fruits and other foods that we'd learned to think of as good and healthy foods that stimulate the immune system. In Dr. Goldberg's theory, such food "literally attacks the brain" in children with autoimmune disorders. The antiviral diet promotes foods rich in protein, including meat, fish, and eggs, and, surprisingly, more processed foods such as white flour and potatoes and other foods that I had considered unhealthy or overly processed. But children with ASD are able to absorb these foods more easily precisely because they are refined and processed. Goldberg's research also emphasizes the common occurrence of viral disorder in children with ASD and recommends both antiviral medication and the removal of foods that feed various herpes viruses, such as the Epstein-Barr virus that we found in Lina's blood shortly after her seizure at three and a half years old.

Any parent of a child with autism will testify that it isn't very easy to evaluate any given treatment. Having a child with autism, or other special needs, often means that there are multiple treatment factors involved at any given time. Evaluating any one remedy often feels like guessing rather than knowing. For a while, it did seem like Lina was doing well with the antiviral diet. She was more expressive, not just requesting things but beginning to comment more on the world around her. She also seemed more able to pay attention to, understand, and follow directions. About a month into the new diet, Lina began to calm down. She didn't scream as much. Soon, she seemed a little less desperate for the very foods that she has always craved with special intensity such as blueberries and strawberries, rice crackers, and nuts. Her gestures and speech seemed increasingly intentional. And she responded more to our questions and limit-setting. Her stimming increased, as when she walked around the playground searching for chewing gum. But her activities didn't seem so frenetic. Jill, the head teacher at Rebecca School, reported that Lina had peacefully sat through the whole *Toy Story* movie during a field trip to the neighborhood movie theatre. Her sleeping also improved.

Tony and I attributed much of Lina's progress to the new diet. In my heart, I thanked God and congratulated my choice of father to my children. Tony and I had screwed up our marriage, but as co-parents and partners in finding Lina, we had become a pretty good team. And Tony's thinking and theorizing and hypothesizing on matters related to Lina's well-being never ends.

His love and appreciation for every crazy little thing she has ever done during her unusual and very action-filled life journey is just as obvious and whole-hearted as his vision for her future. Nothing gets Tony as excited as some new theory that could be helpful to Lina. To spend time with Tony, no matter who you are, is to be presented with long accounts about how he had discovered how large volumes of food made Lina more frenetic or how she shouldn't eat right before bedtime or how she should have meat and potatoes for dinner or how she shouldn't have fruit. Eventually, Tony started to arrange playdates with other families with children with autism symptoms, or with neuro-typical (what others might call "normal") kids who might be willing to play with Lina, while discussing with the other parents the potential remedies for children like Lina. Many nights, Tony sat around with his new girlfriend, frustrating her with his single-minded focus on what to do next for Lina. For miles and miles, months and years, long after she had become too heavy for everyone else to carry, Lina kept getting shoulder rides from Tony, watching New York City go by from behind her papa's big head, feeling safe and comfortable on his broad shoulders.

Throughout our own personal marital challenges, my love for my ex-husband has survived because of his love for my two daughters. Not for a moment did I, Lina, or Elsa doubt that they were at the center of his heart and his life. My little girls never have to doubt that their father will do anything in his power to make them happy. That makes me happy.

With the new Goldberg diet of meat, eggs, potato chips, and Rice Krispies or processed corn flakes with soy milk, Lina's well-being seemed to continue to improve. The teachers at Rebecca School started to make comments about Lina being calmer and more engaged with other children. With her pronounced Spanish accent, Elsa's friend's babysitter, Maria, asked me, "What happened to Lina? She is doing so well!"

Mimmi, one of many people that Tony initially befriended and I eventually adopted, who never says anything she doesn't mean and who comes with a certain inherited Dutch skepticism, started to make frequent observations on Lina's progressive changes. To give Elsa a break from extended subway rides downtown right after her own school days were over, Mimmi offered to let Elsa stay with her and her two sons, Jonas and Oliver, on Thursday afternoons while I went to pick up Lina. Later on Thursdays, we would all meet up in a wooded area of Central Park to fly kites and dip our feet in a hidden spring surrounded by large rocks that the kids could play in. Lina loved these meetings. Every Thursday, regardless of whether I had remembered to prepare Lina for these weekly gatherings, Lina would say, "Go see Mimmi and Jonas," or, "Go see Jonas and Oliver." Mimmi noticed how Lina seemed much more connected, able to listen and answer questions, and stop herself much more effectively when one of us asked her to slow down. She saw how Lina seemed much better able to wait for someone to come with her when she wanted to run off, or tell us when she needed to use the bathroom. There is nothing as exciting as someone else noticing how your children find their way in the world, since my own hopes for Lina sometimes cloud my judgment, making it difficult for me to be certain the progress I notice is real rather than just my wishful thinking.

Lina's old friend Ellen, on one of her family's visits to New York, came into the kitchen one early morning. Lina was already up and at the breakfast table, but upon seeing her old friend, she stood up and the two old friends smiled into each other's eyes and gave each other a hug. Soon, they were both sitting quietly by the table, munching on pancakes just like in the old days. Ellen listened carefully to how Lina was asking for things and talking to me and looked at me with genuine surprise and said, "Lina is so much better! She talks so much more! Was she born with that?"

"No, when Lina was younger she didn't have any trouble finding her words. Remember when you guys used to play together, with your dolls and with the pretend kitchen with all the food toys?"

"I do remember," Ellen said and disappeared into her memories. I turned to Lina, hugged her, and whispered in her ear, "You are so perfect, baby. And you've been finding so many words. You're my little angel."

When Ellen had left the kitchen to play Ariel and Snow White games with Elsa, Lina looked at me, smiled, and referred to the preschool she and Ellen had attended when they were both turning two: "Purple Circle!"

"You remember!" I smiled back.

"Yeah!" Lina confirmed, now smiling broadly.

"You remember how you and Ellen used to go there and play."

"Yeah!"

On Lina's seventh birthday in July 2010, Tony's brother, "Uncle Charlie," came by with a Beyoncé CD that Lina loved. After the corn cake and gingersnap cookies that Lina had ordered for her birthday breakfast, Charlie, who had been observing Lina joining the conversation, answering questions, requesting things, and acting calm and poised, commented on how different she was.

This year was the first year since she turned three that Lina was actually able to enjoy her birthday. At school, as soon as I came through the classroom door to celebrate her, Lina started to sing quickly, "Happy birthday to you, happy birthday to you," anticipating the goodies that couldn't come quickly enough. She sped up the second part of the song to a frenzy without wasting time with any space in between the words in the song: "happy-birthdaytoLinahappybirthdaytoyou!" Lina wasn't too keen on sharing her cinnamon buns with the other kids and teachers in her class. Instead, she pulled the large tray of buns to the space right in front of her and started to chew them down, as quickly as she had just sung her birthday song.

When our friends Anki, Anders, Ellen, and Alfred came over for our second birthday celebration, Lina helped open her own present for the first time in four years. And when one of them turned out to be a beautiful orange, pink, and yellow backpack with a big sunflower on it, at her father's encouragement, she even tried it on! She was fully engaged and participating in the joy of the occasion as well as participating in the rituals of the celebration. First the singing, greeting her with the house decorated in balloons and ribbons, then the dinner, then the cleanup, then more singing and the cake, in this case the cinnamon buns that Lina loves so much, then the blowing out of the candles crammed on one of the buns, then eating, then presents and playing and hanging out. In the past few years, all the little details had been wiped out for the big focus on getting to the CAKE! While that was still important to Lina, it was also clear that she was happy and enjoying having her favorite people around. She remembered her connection with Ellen, at times spontaneously coming up to her and giving her a kiss on the cheek and at other times, just watching her friend sitting next to her on the floor, cutting out patterns in the pile of wrapping paper in front of them. And she didn't scream or even whine once, during the entire evening. The next morning, Lina's first comment was, "Can I please have a birthday!" On her way to school that morning, Lina carried her backpack on her own back for the first time ever.

As we connected Lina's progress to the new diet, we felt it was becoming clear that so many of her problems were directly related to gastrointestinal problems. But while this diet was clearly benefiting Lina, it also seemed to increase the frequency of loose stools and sometimes diarrhea. One summer morning just before Lina's birthday, a social worker from Rebecca School called and informed me that Lina had diarrhea and needed to be picked up from school. Surprised, since Lina had been not been ill and had been her usual, active self that same morning, I called back and asked if there were any other signs of Lina not feeling well or if she had soiled her clothes.

Lina's clothes were clean and she had no fever, but I was told that it was school policy that kids needed to go home when they had diarrhea.

I explained that she'd had diarrhea on and off for the past two months, since we'd started her on the new diet. Gastrointestinal issues such as constipation are extremely common in kids with autism.

"That's just our policy. She needs to go home."

"But can you just hear me out? If Lina needs to go home every time you notice that she has diarrhea or loose stools she would be home all the time! She is not sick. She is just on a diet that is making this happen a little more frequently." (In fact, diarrhea is not necessarily considered to be a negative. It can mean that toxins are exiting a child's system more effectively than in the past.)

"When can you be here?" she insisted.

Tony and I decided to write to the director at the school. The director told us that it would be okay to keep Lina in school if I wrote a note explaining Lina's diet. The next day the same social worker left me two messages stating that a letter from me was not sufficient. I called the director, who wriggled out of it by saying that since in my letter I'd referred to a doctor recommending the diet, he should write another letter. I remember wondering, 'Why shouldn't I refer to the doctor's advice? Did they think I had come up with this diet by myself?' But Tony contacted Dr. Goldberg, who emailed a letter that was approved by the director. In addition, I got a letter from our pediatrician, stating the same correlation between the diet and loose stools. The director was satisfied with Dr. Goldberg's email. The social worker, on the other hand, was still not happy and left me another couple of messages the next day stating that the letter from my pediatrician had the wrong name on it and unless I had "the correct letter, Lina would be sent home and not able to come back until she has one!" Finally, the details were straightened out and Lina was welcomed to stay in school by everyone.

It's no coincidence, I think, that according to Buddhist philosophy, ignorance is a sin. For as long as people believe autism as well as other developmental and neurological challenges to be incurable—originating in some psychodynamically challenging childhood or as something that's inherently wrong in these children's brains, rather than due to environmental toxins in vaccines, paints, and foods, and/or spiritual matters that we have yet to understand along the path of our own enlightenment—parents will beat their heads against walls in facing the lack of understanding in doctors, social workers, teachers, and the general public and we will not change the lives of our children. While nothing is simple and straightforward, and there are many angles from which we can understand and interpret children with autism—including spiritual, psychodynamic, and genetic ones—much current research points in the direction of environmental toxins as well as gastrointestinal issues. It is a relief to a parent as well as for the suffering child when such issues are acknowledged and respected.

Eventually, it turned out, this diet wasn't quite the miracle cure Tony and I had hoped it would be. A few months into the summer, with Lina having been on the diet for most of that winter and spring, during the last couple of weeks at school before the August summer break, Lina's language again became more compromised. Her sleeping patterns again became irregular. Biting reappeared. Screaming resurfaced. Tony and I had to admit that Dr. Goldberg didn't have all the answers, either, at least not for Lina. We reintroduced a more balanced diet, still gluten-, casein-, and sugar-free, but removed the processed foods and reintroduced more fruits and vegetables.

One day, after Lina had gone back to her standard diet, as I was working in my office, Tony called. The background was noisy; he was sitting at a café with a friend, reading from a magazine about allergies. There was hope in his voice. "It says here that 80 percent of all people with schizophrenia suffer from egg allergies. It's the one thing we have never excluded from Lina's diet!" It was true, I couldn't think of any other major foods that we hadn't already tried to exclude from Lina's diet: gluten, casein, sugar, soy, berries, nuts, rice, whole grains (not just the whole grains with gluten), corn . . . the list goes on. But never eggs. I thought about the upcoming week. No school. No distractions. Lina never says no to a friendly egg. She asks for them at least fifty times a day. She gets them, minus most of the egg yolks, which she doesn't like, three times a day. The eggs are complemented with other foods, but they are always on her menu. This egg absence would certainly not go unnoticed by her.

The first week we noticed very little difference on the egg-free diet. But by the second and third week Lina seemed a little calmer, screamed less, and seemed more comfortable in her own skin. Even during Lina's first week back in school in the fall, with many new kids as well as teachers, she seemed calmer. The diminishment in her screaming and crazy running around trying to get her pants off before anyone could stop her, and the fact that biting again stopped, felt like a cool breeze on a hot, humid summer day. Elsa noticed the change instantly. She started to express love and affection for Lina, who would send flashes of a smile in her little sister's direction, so brief that most people would miss them, but for a trained eye like Elsa's, they reinforced the good feeling between them.

Was the egg-free diet the revolutionary breakthrough Tony and I secretly hoped for? No. There were still days when screaming and running around, throwing things, and pulling her clothes off were the major themes. But, whether related to eggs or not, the overall picture was a calmer, more centered Lina. Maybe the protein in eggs was particularly hard for Lina to break down, leading to gastrointestinal pain. Or maybe the poorly processed egg protein created problems in Lina's brain that led to her hyperactivity and screaming. No one really ever knows. Maybe eggs or no eggs have nothing to do with it. But for a while, as long as we could trace an overall improvement in Lina's affect and behavior, eggs were no longer part of her diet. Unfortunately, eventually the benefits of the egg-free diet seemed to fade and we deduced that eggs weren't really the problem.

No sugar and no gluten have stood the test of time. After all the other diets, that is what we returned to. That, and eliminating many of the things that cause Lina stress: traveling on the subway through midtown to school, or being forced through too many difficult transitions on any given day, or suffering through the painful sensation of me brushing through her thick lion's mane of hair each morning.

One day, I asked Tony to take Lina to get her hair cut really short. He would be braver about that than I would have been.

A couple of days after that, a Thursday afternoon after Lina had stayed at Tony's place as she always does on Wednesday nights, I met an altered Lina in the hallway. She looked amazing.

"Who did this one? It's so much better than any haircut she has ever had!" I asked Tony.

"Take a guess," he said cryptically.

"Same place as before, where the kids sit in cars and watch videos?"

"Nope."

After further futile guessing, I heard the story of how he had taken Lina to three different hair places, all claiming they don't cut girls' hair or kids' hair or special girls' hair, only to return to his apartment, place Lina in the bathtub, splash lots of water on her head, and proceed to cut it himself. That took true courage.

For the last couple of years, Tony and I have worked well together with the challenges of having a child who needs much more. In the middle of negotiating our separation agreement, which is the obligatory precursor to divorce in New York, Lina and Elsa remained at the center of our hearts. The connectedness that comes from prioritizing the same thing, being forced to overcome challenges together and loving the same little people, should not be underestimated. For Tony, loving Lina and Elsa includes loving me. For me, watching Tony love Lina and Elsa forces our challenges to the background and inspires me to love and respect him.

CHAPTER NINE

Seizures

It had been a nice Saturday morning in the summer of 2010 and Tony and I and Lina and Elsa were in Central Park with another family of four. Lina was so peaceful. She strolled around the playground without her usual hyperactivity and eventually lay down on a park bench, basking in the sun. Tony and I just stared at her. This was amazing. As Lina was still on Dr. Goldberg's diet, we attributed Lina's revolutionary calm to the diet. Later, we all sat down in an outside café by Sheep's Meadow with our friends. Lina remained seated in her chair, waiting patiently for Tony and me to make up our minds about what foods would be okay for her to eat. It was surreal to see her so peaceful. I felt a sense of happiness and wonder about the normalcy of the situation. This is what it's like for families who don't have hyperactive kids to be out at a café on a Saturday morning. Then Lina came over to my chair and curled up in my lap. That's when I noticed that she was warm. After the outing I took Lina home to Therese, our long-term babysitter who still came to us on most Saturdays.

That Saturday afternoon, I had plans with Derek, a man I had met a few months after moving back to New York. He is a boxer and our first "date" was me showing him how to do yoga. We both spent most of that yoga session lying around on the floor, laughing hysterically. Derek spent most of the rest of his hour resting in child's pose. Being with Derek felt like the most natural thing in the world. It felt like coming home. We had been seeing each other for about a year and a half. We had plans to drive to Connecticut to play beach volleyball with some old volleyball friends of mine. I told Therese to keep giving Lina water and keep her in a cool, air-conditioned place for the rest of the afternoon and keep me updated on how she was doing. An hour later, Therese texted me to let me know Lina's fever was down and she seemed in good spirits, playing at the sensory gym she went to every Saturday afternoon during this period.

My small leased Honda Accord, packed with food, a hungry boyfriend, his two sisters, one sister's partner, and me, was on its way. Our feet had barely touched the sand before my cell phone rang. Derek had already jokingly predicted that we would have to turn back because of my daughter. The previous Saturday afternoon, Derek and his teenage son and one of the sisters had come with me to the same beach. That time, our trip was cut short because of Tony ending up in the hospital with kidney stones. This Saturday was a re-run. But this time, it was Lina.

We ended up fighting about going back. Maybe Derek was tired of taking his family to the beach only to have to rush back because of my family's emergencies. All I knew was that Lina seemed to have had a second seizure when on the bus with Therese and was now on her way to the hospital. That was all I needed to know.

"Get in the car or don't! Please make a decision! I'm leaving. NOW!"

"Come with me in the car for two minutes; let's talk about it," Derek said, significantly more level-headed than myself.

"I don't have two minutes!" I yelled with the Buddha necklace that Derek had given to me flying around my neck, and then, surprising myself, I added, "And just so you know, I want you to come with me. I need you!"

Not knowing anything about what state Lina was in, if she had had more seizures, if she was conscious, if she was in pain and if this seizure would take her further away from us, I was completely oblivious to the fact that my old beach-volleyball friends, standing twenty-five yards away already on the court, were watching me have an increasingly loud screaming match with the boyfriend they had not yet met, no more than two years after they witnessed my marriage with Tony fall apart on that very same beach. All I could tend to at that moment was my own fury about minute after minute going by without me being on my way to my daughter who was now on *her* way to the hospital. After further disgrace, we all ended up in the car, back to New York.

Tony didn't answer his cell phone but Derek helped me track down the right ER and the right nurse who was in the middle of treating Lina. She told me that Lina's temperature was 105 degrees, and I told her that according to our babysitter, who, coincidentally, had been with Lina during both seizures, Lina's reactions during both incidents were very similar in nature. Like last time, Lina had first seemed very weak, with her legs folding under her, and then had some minor body spasms, followed by being out of touch, staring without seeing. The nurse let me speak with the doctor since I was hoping to convince someone to put Lina on an EEG immediately to see if this time we could trace the seizure activity more effectively. It turned out not to be possible, but we had no problem establishing that an overnight EEG was called for and should be arranged.

Walking into the ER and seeing my little girl already recovered enough to fight the nurse over swallowing the fever-reducing Motrin, I felt so grateful. Lina was okay. Elsa was okay. Nothing else was important. Life lets us see this now and then, I think, because as much as we might believe we have our priorities straight, we so easily get sidetracked and distracted. But now, with my girl in my arms, breathing peacefully, all was well in my world.

After the seizure episode, Lina lost some ground. She seemed to struggle even more to find her words. Her voice seemed more monotone for a while and she slipped away from interactions more readily.

A couple of months later, I came into the bedroom where my two girls were spread out on the two queen-sized futons on the floor. I had been watching a late-night movie on my computer, and was looking forward to lying down, draping a bathrobe over myself so as not to wake anyone up by pulling on the blanket. Before drifting off to sleep, I registered a strange smell but in my drowsy state I picked the path of least resistance and moved further into sleep. Half an hour later, I heard Lina coughing, and then that other sound, the sound of vomiting and a weak whining coming from Lina. I sat up, quickly picked up Elsa, put her on a small mattress in her play area in the living room, and then went back to Lina. She was surrounded by vomit. I picked her up, rinsed her off, re-dressed her, wrapped her in a blanket, and put her on the couch in the playroom. I went back to the bedroom and turned the light on. Both beds and large portions of the wall were covered with vomit. Everything—sheets, mattress covers, blankets and pillows and clothes—had to be rinsed and sorted for laundry. I washed the wall, working fast, hoping to be back by Lina's side before the next round. I put Elsa back in the cleaned-up bedroom, closed the door behind her, and arranged clean towels all around Lina in preparation for what was coming. Around six in the morning, Lina's vomiting slowed down. By then, Elsa had moved into the playroom with us, sleeping soundly at the other end of the couch, her feet touching mine for security and reassurance that she wasn't alone.

It was Thanksgiving Day. We had plans to go to Tony's sister's apartment for dinner. A little before noon, Sean came to take Elsa out to the playground while I stayed next to Lina, making sure she kept sipping water and softly talking and singing for her. It's so unusual to have Lina so calm and available. I looked into her eyes, played soft songs from our CDs for her, and talked to her in a slow, soothing voice. She looked at me with her big, blue eyes and pulled my arm closer around her on the couch. I picked up some books and loved the feeling of Lina's attentive listening to the stories. She was too tired, too weakened by last night's sickness to be driven away by her own restless, sensory needs. So she just stayed there, listening to my reading one book after the other.

It was around that time that Lina suddenly turned warm. She started to shiver. I put another blanket on her. She stared out into the empty space in front of her and began to shake. She tipped her head in toward her body and curled up in a fetal position on the couch and kept shaking. Saliva began to drip out of the right side of her mouth and she seemed to have lost control of the muscles in her mouth. I stared at her as she continued to shake, not violently, but in small, continuous tremors, and her eyes no longer met mine but stared past me, experiencing something, somewhere where I could not follow. Her lips turned blue. Momentarily, the shaking stopped. Then it started up again, followed by the same drooling and loss of eye contact. I began to throw things into a bag and put a pull-up diaper on Lina just in case she lost control of her bladder and bowels. Slowly, Lina regained consciousness and as after her previous seizures, her face and her body seemed deprived of every ounce of energy. I called Tony to let him know that I would take a cab to the nearest ER and dressed Lina in clothes that would keep her as warm and comfortable as possible on the way there. Somehow, Tony was in my apartment within ten minutes. Together we walked out onto the street with Lina motionless in my arms, jumped in a cab, and were on our way.

We drove to the hospital with which Lina's neurologist was affiliated, hoping to coordinate Lina's inpatient and outpatient treatments. We spent a couple of hours in the ER, getting blood tests done with Lina screaming at the top of her lungs and with four people, including me and Tony, holding her down. We tried to get an MRI but failed miserably since Lina wouldn't remain still no matter how masterful the combination of belts and thick, cotton blankets intended to keep her in one place for a few seconds at a time. Sedated MRIs weren't an option during the holidays, we were told. In the middle of all this, Tony and I managed to have a minor argument about how we are to talk to each other about our significant others. But, as usual, in the face of Lina's difficulties, our lives simply didn't allow for much ongoing disagreement. While the hours ticked by at the hospital, Elsa was celebrating Thanksgiving at her aunt and uncle's house. Aunt Jennifer was impressed by Elsa's passion for turkey and when I called my little friend on the phone she wanted to get off quickly to continue the Peter Pan game she was engaged in with her cousin Finn, whom Elsa had rediscovered with increasing enthusiasm since our move back to New York.

Another couple of hours later it was decided that Lina would be admitted to the hospital for a seventy-two-hour EEG. Since she had just endured a stomach virus, she would not be allowed to leave her room. It would be mostly me and her in that room for seventy-two hours. I wondered how that would be possible. The first night's challenge was solved with mellowing medication. That made the second round of blood tests easier on everyone and facilitated the EEG technician's challenge of attaching the leads to Lina's head with clay, which was used as a replacement for the much stronger-smelling glue they used for more compliant patients. Miraculously, Lina slept through most of the long process. Minutes after the technician's departure, I was asleep in the folding chair next to Lina's bed. A few hours later, I woke up. Not because of anything Lina did. She slept peacefully throughout the night while my own stomach lurched, and I spent the next few hours running back and forth between my folding chair and the bathroom, hoping none of the nurses would detect my virus and send me home.

By the following afternoon, I felt my strength coming back to me via a cup of peppermint tea that I had asked Tony to bring me when he came to visit. Tony stayed for most of the day at the hospital. Elsa went from a playdate with her friend Isabella to another round of playing with her cousin Finn, until Tony brought her back home to his place. When Tony went to get Elsa, Lina and I sat around in our two giant folding chairs next to the window that faced the East River, eating slowly, cutting paper, me drawing something and asking Lina questions about it and then handing it to her to cut into small pieces. With the occasional interruption by a nurse or a doctor checking in on us for a few minutes, trying to coordinate tests and letting us know that nothing remarkable had yet showed up on the EEG, Lina and I had the kind of peace one can only experience away from home, away from the noise of everyday life. We looked into each other's eyes and said little things to each other now and then. It was still. The third day, Elsa came by. At first excited by the new toys Lina had received, Elsa soon became moody, her feelings about being left behind at Thanksgiving beginning to surface. And the next morning, when Lina was back home after her hospital stay, Elsa woke up in an even darker mood.

"You want to talk about it?" I offered.

"No! . . . I am angry!"

"Mm, want to tell me more?"

"No!"

"You're showing me instead. . . . It must not have been so much fun to be left behind when me and Papa took Lina to the hospital."

Elsa looked up at me, then marched into Lina's playroom and started to move things around. She didn't throw things. She created disorder in a very neat way. She took the tablecloth from the little table and threw it on the floor. She carefully lifted the chairs and turned them upside down. She dumped the teddy bear on the floor as well. The candle also ended up on the floor as well as the couch pillow.

"You're showing me how it felt to be left behind."

"I'm done now," she said, looking relieved. "I'm cleaning up."

"I'll help you."

"Mama, I love you."

"And I love you, my dear. More than you could ever imagine."

Lina's doctor recommended medication to stop any further, potentially damaging, seizures—2.5 ml of Depakote (Depakene) syrup. Sweet enough for Lina not to spit it out. Sweet enough to re-create the yeast in her mouth that makes her laugh uncontrollably and become hyper and more inclined to scream at the top of her lungs. This in spite of the fact that Depakote, in addition to safeguarding against further seizures, also addresses dramatic mood changes in individuals with bipolar disorders. Though, as it turns out, not only did this medication fail to calm Lina down, it also failed to prevent further seizures.

On Tuesday night, between Christmas and New Year's, Lina had another seizure. That, too, was fever induced. With our Sean away for the holidays, I had dropped Lina off at Tony's so I could see a couple of clients before picking her up again for the special one-on-one evening she and I had every Tuesday. But as I was walking out the door of Tony's apartment, Lina, who had a cold and a mild fever, curled up in the bed and started to shake. In less than a minute, her lips had turned blue and her eyes stared off into those unreachable places. We waited for a few minutes. The shaking stopped and her lip color returned to normal. She slept for a little while, while I called my clients to cancel. Soon, Lina seemed almost back to normal. We stayed there for another hour before I took Lina with me for a piggy-back ride home. According to our Tuesday night tradition, Elsa was staying over at Tony's and Lina and I had our special night with just the two of us. Lina and I had a peaceful evening together and she fell asleep at her usual time around ten or ten thirty, but woke up again at one thirty in the morning and stayed up until seven.

While Lina stays up like this once or twice a week, I now wondered if there was something about the recent seizure that made it more difficult for her to relax enough to sleep through the night. I also wondered, as her new neurologist seemed to believe, if Lina, rather than having an atypical version of autism, in fact was challenged with an atypical seizure disorder. Or, rather than subtracting one of her potential diagnoses, should we just add another one? Each year, our questions about Lina kept multiplying. Each year, I tried to learn to accept all the unanswered questions while at the same time not give up on broadening my understanding of what was happening to Lina. As we lay in the dark, watching the night hours turn into early morning, Lina, with her head on my arm, singing and self-talking about all the interesting things she would like to have for breakfast, I wondered how many mothers of seven-year-olds have this opportunity for wordless, timeless closeness with their growing school children? What could ever compare to Lina's soulful smiles so deeply rooted in her being and uncontaminated by words and expectations? It was all worth it, I told myself as I rolled into the shower to get ready for the challenge of getting Lina out of bed and on her way to school.

Spurred by these febrile seizures, Tony and I began the process of attaining Medicaid for Lina so that we could go all the way in our quest for more answers. While neither of us wanted to put Lina through more invasive testing than what was necessary, we wanted to pursue genetic testing since the developmental pediatrician who evaluated Lina at the Children's Neurodevelopment Center in Rhode Island thought we needed to rule out atypical Rett syndrome, a disorder with later onset of developmental challenges brought on by deceleration of head growth around the age of five and including stereotyped movement like hand-wringing, loss of social engagement, impaired language. This wonderful and empathetic pediatrician, like many others, didn't feel certain of the autism diagnosis.

A psychiatric evaluation was done by the psychiatrist at Sick Kids need Involved People (SKIP) of New York, an organization that helps parents of children with special needs deal with issues such as insurance and child care. The somber psychiatrist asked Lina to identify objects in a book while Lina preferred to explore the hallway outside the examining room. "So, Ms. Hjalmarsson, you have absolutely no control over your daughter, do you?" Retaliating is never advisable but nevertheless I could not let the statement go by without responding. "My daughter is more likely to stay in the room if you volunteer a little smile." The rest of the evaluation was conducted over the phone, with me trying the best I could to account for Lina's functioning and development.

The envelope with the completed evaluation lay unopened for a couple of days before I sat down to read it. Turns out, I had good reasons for my trepidation:

Lina Lyons is a lovely, 6 year 10 month old female with a history of Autism. She continues to display significant deficits in many areas of functioning, specifically sensory and language processing, cognitive functioning, social relatedness, attention, and reciprocal play. She cannot be tested with standardized instruments appropriate for her age, but her cognitive delays are significant and comparable to the Moderate range of mental retardation. Her adaptive behavior is equally diminished, as her scores on the VABS II show significant deficits in all domains as well as the composite score. Although her mother has seen recent improvement in her functioning, and continues to provide her daughter with the maximum opportunities for growth and learning, Lina's condition is likely to last indefinitely.

I sat there on the couch, staring at the blurring words of a stranger, determining my daughter's future. Will the grief ever stop? Grief and happiness are strange companions, both so real and true in the context of Lina. The next morning, I woke up with the thought of having another child. Elsa needed a sibling to share the responsibility of caring for and loving Lina when Tony and I were no longer around. "Who should be the father?" I thought, watching my own desperation with a sad, internal smile. What sane divorced forty-five-year-old mother of two, one with autism, has these thoughts? Maybe the fact that Tony and I were almost forty when we had Lina was a contributing factor to her autism? What if the next kid has special needs, too? How would that be for supporting Elsa? Maybe I should adopt? I kept watching my thoughts. Then Elsa and Lina and I made scones. Then I took Elsa to a sibling group. Then I did yoga. And then I was back to being the luckiest mother the sun had ever touched.

The truth is no one had any idea of what was going on with Lina. Speculations were as varied as Lina's behavior on any given day. Atypical Rett syndrome? Atypical, late-onset autism? Developmental language disorder? Sensory processing disorder? Landau-Kleffner syndrome? Childhood disintegrative disorder? Neuro-immune dysfunction? Mental retardation? Seizure disorder? Viruses? After all the expertise that had come Lina's way, we were no closer to the answer than we had been three years earlier, when it all began to unravel.

Lina was scheduled to have an MRI under anesthesia on February 25, 2011. The night before and the morning of, Elsa had a fever and vomited. She had been at a music and theater winter-break camp at Lucy Moses School, and today parents were invited to see the kids perform. Today was also Elsa's dear cousin Finn's birthday party. She would have to miss both. At the very least, with Elsa being sick and facing so much disappointment that day, I wanted to be by her side. But we had been waiting months for this scheduled MRI for Lina. Life involves so much compromise. With heavy steps I left a very disappointed Elsa with a babysitter to take Lina to her MRI. Over the phone, I tried to explain to Elsa that even though I wasn't able to be there to comfort her when she was sick, my thoughts and my heart were just as much with her as with Lina. This is not an easy thing to convey to a child who has a sibling with special and intense needs. But Elsa works so hard at processing all the challenges in her life and to walk through her life as a whole and happy person. She welcomes every opportunity to receive what she needs to find balance in her own life.

Lina did okay. She was very hungry and restless the whole morning as she wasn't allowed to eat or drink prior to the MRI. We were about to put Lina through yet another invasion. In order to learn more about what was going on with her, we were inflicting potential danger on her. Tony and I were tortured by this and on our way to the hospital, we walked right back into the place of hostility and pain that had ended our relationship. I decided to walk ahead to avoid having Lina be in the middle of our difficulties. Encapsulated by that old feeling of panic and rage, I started to run down the street. I couldn't do anything else. Just run. It was as if every painful past memory, every impossible situation, every terrifying experience and excruciating loss from early childhood to adulthood was encapsulated in that moment and I thought, *This is the day when I lose it.* I glanced sideways, the uncontrollable running taking me closer to the medical clinics near the New York University hospital where Lina would have her MRI. One of the clinics had glass doors; outside two EMS trucks were parked. There were nurses and other people inside the clinic looking out at me running down the street. I don't know if I was screaming. It was all a blur. I could see in their faces that they knew I was falling apart. When everything seemed its darkest, my phone rang. It was Derek. Our relationship had ended and I hadn't talked to him for months, but now, hearing his voice, I cried into the phone until I felt like I could breathe normally. The comfort of knowing that somehow, even though we were no longer together, we still had some kind of intuitive connection that had very little to do with words, calmed me down. I found Tony and Lina and walked with them into the crowded hospital lobby.

When Lina finally was led into the room for her MRI with nurses holding a mask over her mouth and nose while others were restraining her strong, flailing arms and legs, I felt just as helpless on her behalf as I had during her previous MRI, three years earlier. It seemed like we were violating the trust that we had worked so hard to build. Tony's expression mirrored my feelings. And Lina appeared to agree. As soon as she was able to form sounds after the anesthesia began to lift, her body began to writhe in anger and her screaming was soon in full bloom, completely commanding the attention of the entire MRI unit. She screamed, and then ate some blueberries with unsteady hands and a mouth that was still drooping from numbness, eyes only half opened. Then she threw up. Then she peed all over the floor, the armchair, her clothes, and shoes. Then she screamed for another half hour, until we decided that even though she was unhappy, her strength and vital signs were not in question. With her arms tightly wrapped around my neck and with Tony quietly by my side I carried her out on the street to look for a cab. As Tony and I were standing there with Lina I noted that whatever anger had been between us had now passed, and in my bag were the tubes of blood drawn while Lina was knocked out, which I would deliver to the genetics department at another NYC hospital after the weekend. Tony was there, alongside me, fighting for our daughter's recovery. In spite of our difficulties, we would both always be there, side by side, trying to help our daughter.

A couple of weeks later, the social worker from the genetics department at New York Presbyterian Hospital informed us that Lina's results for the Rett syndrome testing were normal. So were the microarray test results. The Chromosomal Microarray Analysis (CMA) screens the entire genome, which makes it possible to pick up and establish subtle genetic mutations across the genome, increasing the likelihood of finding abnormalities that other genetic testing may not detect. Since genetic abnormalities associated with autism traditionally have been difficult to measure, this new microarray analysis, at that time, was the best genetic test for autism. The following week, Dr. LaJoise, the same neurologist who had examined Lina years ago, reported that nothing unusual had shown up on Lina's MRI.

But despite not having a quantitative way to measure it, something had definitely changed after Lina's last seizure. At first, I just viewed it as another step in her development. And maybe it was a kind of self-assertion. And maybe emotions that had been in hiding were surfacing and now triggered dramatic tantrums. Actually, the word "tantrums" does not suffice to describe the kind of catastrophic emotional and physical events that Lina began to experience on an increasingly frequent basis. "Earthquakes" or "volcanoes" would be more descriptive of the kind of explosions that Lina started to experience. Lina's teachers began to report them as well. Her head teacher called me one day after one of these episodes, telling me how Lina's despair and emotional tumult had moved her to the point that she was crying alongside Lina. I thanked her for the emotional honesty involved in that interaction and we agreed to keep trying to support Lina through these storms the best we could. I felt convinced that the storm would eventually pass.

A month went by and nothing much changed. In fact, it got even worse. Lina would start screaming as we started to eat dinner and would try to tilt the whole dinner table over. She would try to throw whatever foods she could grab before I stopped her. She would tear down the mirror from the wall. She would bite, kick, and scream so loud that my ears hurt. When she was out in public, screaming in this way, people would get furious. Or they would laugh or want to call a doctor or condemn me for not stopping her. I would screen out everyone else but Lina the best I could and try to focus on maintaining a peaceful, calm presence. No overreacting. No attempts to try to make her stop screaming. No giving her what she wanted so that she would stop screaming. Keeping her safe, offering a word or two to describe what she seemed to be feeling, and waiting it out—those were my only options. But the episodes continued. I began to feel burdened. On edge. I wanted to yell back and make her stop. And sometimes I did. But most of all I wanted to put the judgmental observers in their place. And sometimes I did.

Lina and I were on the street outside our apartment building. Lina had asked for potato chips. I had said yes, not a problem, we can eat potato chips with dinner. But Lina was confused. She kept yelling that she wanted potato chips while I kept telling her, "You'll have them, baby, it's okay, we are going to have them as soon as we get home." But Lina was inconsolable. We got to our lobby. Lina kept screaming. A young man in his twenties, who was visiting someone on the first floor of my building, opened the apartment door, looked at us, clearly upset about the situation, and without a word slammed the door behind him with all his power. Lina kept screaming. I took her hand and went to knock on the door. The young man and his friend opened the door.

"She has autism. What's your problem?" I said, looking straight into his eyes.

But of course I didn't know what was going on with my daughter. A few nights later, with more screaming and explosions, kicking and destroying things, yet another swollen bite mark on my shoulder, more tears and a sense of being depleted, and Lina regressing back to being incontinent both day- and nighttime, I thought about the Depakote, Lina's anti-seizure medication. Maybe Lina's breakdowns were not so much related to self-assertion as some kind of discomfort caused by this drug? Reading online about the side effects of Depakote, I found what I was looking for. Among the common side effects were mood swings, behavioral changes, anxiety, and confusion. It was also clearly stated that Depakote should not be taken by anyone with brain development issues and/or gastrointestinal issues. As I picked up Lina and Elsa that evening from Tony's house, I thought about how Lina's seizures, ever since the summer, had all been fever induced. Why not just treat Lina's fever more assertively with ibuprofen and see if we could prevent further seizures that way? Tony instantly agreed. The two neurologists involved in prescribing the Depakote were both on vacation, and the doctor on call did not return our call.

So we took Lina off of Depakote. It wasn't the gentle, textbook, tapering-off process recommended for most psychotropic medications. It was instant. Neither Tony nor I could face giving Lina any more Depakote. The result was immediate. The first thing I noticed was that Lina started to smile. It was as if she felt happy to be back to herself. The screaming instantly subsided. The second night after we stopped Depakote, Lina woke up dry. Daytime accidents immediately stopped. She seemed more connected both to herself and those around her. The experience left me with a promise to myself to always thoroughly research anything that is recommended by anyone from the medical community or beyond and never let anyone make me think that I don't have a choice in what medication and/or treatment I subject my children to. And I also promised myself to try more natural remedies should Lina have more seizures. Tony sent me a link to a natural product called Epi-Still. It would "promote complete nervous system health . . . help maintain neuron health and neural connections . . . encourage brain stability and harmony" and many more wonderful things. I was excited and ready to buy three bottles of Epi-Still and another with the "Neuro-Toner" that went with it, when I realized that neither the woman on the phone promoting the remedy nor the description on the Epi-Still website could, or would, account for the actual ingredients. "A combination of selected herbal ingredients" was as far as I got.

I went to my local health-food store owner instead, and after a half-hour discussion with him and borrowing a book describing the natural remedy GPC (L-alphaglycerophosphatidylcholine, also known as choline alfoscerate, derived from lecithin and also found in human breast milk), I decided to give it a try. Prescribed to a wide range of patients with brain issues, including very successful and extensive clinical trials on Alzheimer's patients, GPC had also been found to improve communication, social interactions, mood, cognition, and focus in children with autism.

I considered this a kind of substitute for the Depakote, to help calm down Lina's brain and raise the threshold for seizures. After a week and a half of her taking GPC, everyone involved with Lina's care, from teachers at school to babysitters (without knowing about the new medication), commented on her increased acting-out behavior. I consulted Dr. Darren Lynch, the biomedical DAN doctor who had been very helpful in administering tests and trying out various diets and biomedical treatments for Lina from the onset of her autism. Dr. Lynch first recommended quercetin. While quercetin is mostly known for its ability to provide cardiovascular support and as a dietary antioxidant, it also has anti-inflammatory and antihypertensive properties that are thought to relax brain activity and therefore increase the threshold for seizures. Lina again reacted with increased hyperactivity. So we switched to carnosine, which, Dr. Lynch explained, is a membrane-stabilizing antioxidant that could help Lina calm down in general and in her brain in particular, helping to raise the seizure threshold. Carnosine did seem to work. Lina did not have any additional seizures while on this medication.

CHAPTER TEN

Predicaments

Having fun with someone who constantly wants to do repetitive things and who has trouble maintaining focus and engagement for very long takes a bit of imagination. The safest way of giving Lina a good time is to take her to the beach. Summer in New York City is hot and humid. The beach is the perfect antidote for everyone. On one Monday in July, I just wasn't looking forward to taking Lina and Elsa to playgrounds in Central Park, or having dinner in our hot kitchen while sweat dripped down our foreheads and spines. So I took Elsa and Sean with me in the car that Tony was leasing to pick up Lina at her summer school. Normally it takes an hour to get from the Upper West Side to Westport. "Our" beach in Westport is less crowded than most public beaches and the beautiful wooden playground right next to the beach has the kind of tire swings that sustain Lina's attention for up to twenty minutes at a time. Today we sat in the car for three and a half hours, starting out at two o'clock and getting to the beach at five thirty. Lina had spiced up the monotonous traffic jam by quietly throwing her brand new shoes out the window. I had soon noticed it and glanced back on the shoulder of the highway and actually saw one of the shoes. But right in front of me, I spotted a policeman and, unsure of the rules, I made a mental note of the nearby exit and figured I would pick the shoes up on the way back. Seconds before we turned into the parking lot next to the beach, Elsa, who often gets carsick, threw up all over herself and all over the car seat and the floor in front of her. Trying desperately to keep a positive spin on our increasingly challenging outing, I heard myself saying, "Oh, that's okay, don't worry, that's great, really!" *Great?* Who did I think I was kidding? Was Elsa suddenly going to think it was great to have thrown up all over herself because I said so? I smiled to myself. I actually didn't have to make it great when it wasn't.

Parking the car, I realized I hadn't brought any extra clothes for Elsa, and only one bathing suit between the two girls (Elsa had taken hers out of the bag for a fitting in front of the mirror) and no underwear for myself. And what was I wearing? My bathing suit. Elsa was very unhappy. At five years old, at the peak of her princess stage, she was not at all impressed with my idea of jumping right into the water with her clothes on. I made my decision. Plagued with the kind of guilt only a mother can have when she knows she is treating her children unethically,

I gave Elsa Lina's bathing suit and put the puked-on clothing on Lina. My sweet Lina didn't mind, which made it both better and worse. And what definitely made everything more complicated was that five minutes into the swimming, Lina got stung by jellyfish. Not badly, but badly enough for her to actually get up from the water and whimper. But Lina recovered quickly and was soon in the water again, with me anxiously searching the water all around the girls for more of the unpleasant and even dangerous creatures.

An hour later, we were on our way back again, Elsa in only her underwear, me without (I had on a T-shirt and shorts, but I'm not one of those women from the sixties who walks around regularly without bras or inhibitions) and Lina, well, Lina had an economy bag of potato chips in her lap so whatever the aftermath of the minor jellyfish stings she might have had, the discomfort of it was overruled by the pleasure of crunching on something salty.

Approaching the exit where Lina had dropped her shoes, I quietly formulated my plan. I would find a safe place to pull over on the side of the highway, jump out of the car, cross the highway, and pick up Lina's shoes. I figured Lina's nice, brand-new fifty-dollar shoes were of no use to anyone discarded by the roadside, and were only a fast hundred-yard dash away. I spotted first one, then the other, twenty yards apart. After scooping them up and congratulating myself, I looked up to see a police car pulling up behind our car. A policeman approached the car, spoke to Sean, then stomped down his side of the highway in my direction. Damn! I crossed the highway while he made wild, angry gestures to the oncoming cars to slow down and stop to enable me to cross. Not good. He clearly was focused on demonstrations of rescuing me from myself and my own bad judgment. That was only the beginning. Back at my car, he lectured me about acting responsibly, taking into account that I had young ones depending on me, etc., etc. I was never in danger but this was not the time or the place to be contrary. Instead, I took a more humble approach, but that didn't do it either. My daughter's shoes were now worth $125, including the $75 ticket handed to me. Oh, and I was now officially granted a criminal record for reckless behavior in traffic. I guess I was lucky that the flustered policeman wasn't angry enough to throw the shoes back to the other side just to further prove his point.

"F---ing prick!" I let out, temporarily unable to censor myself in front of my children, as the policeman climbed back into his car. *Why do I try so hard, when everything goes to shit?* I asked myself, this time inwardly, without further exposing Lina and Elsa to my personal frustration. But Elsa, seeing the tears that started rolling down my cheeks, in her usual, nurturing spirit, said, "Mama, I love you."

"Thank you, baby, I know you do. Thanks for saying that. I love you, too."

"Mama, why are you sad?"

"Oh, I'm just frustrated about the ticket. It's really not a big deal. You know me, I may get upset but soon I forget all about it and we'll all be laughing about the whole thing."

"I know how you feel."

"Do you, baby?"

"Yes, you see, once something like this happened to me, too, I was . . . ehrr, kind of . . . well . . ."

Was that my five year-old talking? Where did this little curly haired cherub come from? She would say, "I come from God," and that was as far as I got in my own speculations about her origins.

Soon enough, the little Honda Accord was filled with bubbly laughter and jokes about my newly acquired criminal record, Lina's expensive shoes, and the policeman's ill-concealed frustration about my highway expedition. Sweet Sean tried to convince me to let him pay half my ticket since he had agreed with me that it should be no problem dashing across to pick up those shoes. Loyal and supportive as he is, he then proceeded to give Lina and Elsa and me a long speech about how the policeman's decision to write me a ticket was poorly founded and made no sense. Elsa got caught up in her own reasoning about whether or not I should have gotten the ticket, whether or not I should have known not to do this, and what we could all learn from the experience. For her, the most obvious lesson was that Mamas should not run on the highway but instead call the police so they could help pick up the shoes. I learned that one, too, but it was nice to have the useful part of the day reiterated by someone other than myself.

Susan, mother to eleven-year-old Rebecca, who was also a student at Rebecca School, never hesitates to make a joke about herself or her situation. And when she mocks herself for getting pissed off at her daughter still peeing in the bed or feeling embarrassed or panicked when her loving, good-natured daughter walks up to little babies in the playground and wants to touch them or twirl their hair, you can see how well this ability to see humor in everything works for her. Her stories are almost always accompanied by a deep belly laugh that relieves the tension both in her and everyone around her.

"I laugh during the day and cry at night," she told me, and then went on to describe a kind of hole puncher with various patterns, flowers, stars, and hearts, that Lina, who loves cutting things with scissors, might appreciate. Rebecca and Susan and her husband, Ryan, and their younger daughter Rachel had started coming by our house on Saturdays to see if Rebecca and Lina could find a way to socialize and to give opportunities for Elsa and Rachel to hang out while the rest of us ate, made jokes, and compared notes about our crazy lives. Elsa and Rachel had made an instant connection with each other at a group where the siblings of students at Rebecca School meet to try out their sisters' and brothers' sensory gym, eat pizza, and talk about what it is like to deal with their siblings' unpredictable screaming and laughing, strange sleep habits, and ways of talking and playing that are so different from typical kids.

Before deciding upon playdates at my house, Susan and I optimistically came up with the not-so-intelligent idea of taking Rebecca and Lina to a busy downtown playground. Too distracted, Rebecca and Lina did not exchange a single word with each other. Rebecca went into the sprinklers and Lina started her usual running around, climbing everything and looking for chewing gum on the ground. For a few seconds, I managed to motivate Lina to go on the tire swing, but by the time Susan had gotten Rebecca to agree to go on, Lina was long gone. Lina likes chasing games. With a twist. Just chasing her isn't enough. There has to be some excitement to the game. I imagine in Lina's head it's something like, "I'm going to pull my pants down. Then your face is going to look funnier and more colorful and you will chase me down with more passion." And it works. Because if you don't chase her down when she is running around official places with a bare butt, half of the population of Manhattan will come and stare at you. Innumerable bystanders will offer plenty of advice and opinions even when you're actively pursuing an exhilarated child, but at least you will miss most of what they say. Silence is much underrated in this country. Susan knows this. She wouldn't offer any advice in those situations and her quiet acceptance and relaxed attitude meant so much more to me than a hundred well-meaning comments. And when Rebecca squatted down next to the sprinklers, still in her bathing suit, all I offered were some tissues to wipe up the mess. It was a little while after that, with Lina and Rebecca still not having exchanged even brief glances in each other's direction, that I decided to put Lina, who now was running around stark naked, laughing hysterically, on the back of my bike and go home.

It's all relative. Overall, over time, Lina's pace has slowed down dramatically. She listens when you ask her to wash her hands or put her dinner plate in the sink instead of in the garbage. Most of the time, she is not so distracted that she cannot answer questions and she puts more and more feeling and meaning into her words. And, most importantly, she almost never runs away. A couple of months after our move back to New York City, Valerie and I looked at each other and realized that someone had forgotten to lock the door to our apartment and Lina had snuck out. Dashing down the stairs, taking one staircase each while leaving Elsa behind with a fast "We'll be back in a minute, don't worry," we met in the lobby with increasing panic, still without a sign of Lina. I sent Valerie outside the building while running up the stairs one more time with the intention of searching each floor. On my way down the stairs after one more frenetic search and another hasty reassurance to Elsa, I came to the second floor and noticed that the door to apartment B was wide open.

I got closer and heard my daughter's wild laughter from inside. The middle-aged man who lives in that apartment with his wife, whom I had recently met in the laundry room, came out into the hallway. He looked puzzled and smiled at me, gesticulating for me to come into his living room. I followed him and saw Lina, stark naked, laughing and screaming with delight, jumping up and down on the couple's couch. Her clothes were spread around their living room floor. I picked up my excited daughter, noticed with gratefulness that the man was still smiling, and excused ourselves as quickly as I could, fully aware that little Elsa was left alone upstairs. From then on, my good-humored neighbor made funny little references to my unruly daughter whenever we ran into each other in the lobby and elevator until one day I teasingly said, "Okay, so she jumped on your couch. We've been over this a few times. Many things, believe me, many interesting things have happened since then. So let's move on, shall we?" It was soon after that conversation that this neighbor presented himself to me in the lobby as the owner of the building. My only comfort was that somehow, the man was still smiling.

It was Saturday morning, 8:17 a.m. I was standing in the kitchen, newly awake and not yet showered in oversized shorts and a tank top making coffee before doing some yoga, seeing my nine o'clock client, and picking up my angels at Tony's place, where both of them stay on Friday nights. The downstairs doorbell rang. Somehow, I had forgotten about my 8:15 a.m. client. Before our life was turned upside down by the changes in Lina,

I was an extremely organized individual and a devoted therapist. It wasn't just that I would never forget about the people I had taken on or their hours. I would only rarely reschedule their sessions. I would dream about them, think about them, discuss them in supervision, and be peaceful and ready every time they walked in through my door.

Now, I often come flying down the street on my bike after having dropped one or two of my girls off somewhere. Now, most of the time, I walk in through the lobby together with my clients, with disintegrating sandals and unbrushed hair, out of breath and with a piece of bagel or a coffee in one hand and my bike in the other. These days, I reschedule all the time and, like this morning, I often simply forget about appointments. But I've developed skills in becoming ready when the moment suddenly requires it. My 8:15 client never found out that I had just climbed out of bed. I put my hair in a ponytail, splashed some water on my face, jumped into a shirt and slacks, and opened the door with a smile, soon sharing my morning coffee with him.

Once my clients manage through the initial disarray and are here, right in front of me, I'm with them, fully present and happy to be there with them. But when they are not standing before me, life with Lina and Elsa overshadows everything else. Things have gotten better, but if I don't concentrate, there is still a chance that Lina could run right into the street and be instantly killed. Or, less dramatically, if I don't watch her every move, she could pick up and eat a piece of chewing gum that might have belonged to someone with hepatitis B. That's what mothers of one-year-olds worry about, but their kids are not as fast or as smart or as goal-oriented as Lina. My daughter enters the playground with an intention to find chewing gum and candy dropped on the ground. She claims that she wants to swing because she knows that if she says she wants to go to the playground with the most candy on the ground, I will say no and we will go someplace else.

On that particular morning of the forgotten 8:15 client, Lina and Elsa and I did go to the playground after my two appointments. And Lina liked the one we chose for the wrong reasons. Ten minutes into it, I decided to find a different playground, with less candy and chewing gum on the ground. Lina was not happy with this decision. I took her hand and we had gotten to the sidewalk outside the playground gates when she threw her shoes off and sat down on the ground. Disappointments are often torture for Lina, but I just felt unable to face another minute of chasing her around to prevent her from putting something chewy and colorful in her mouth.

"Lina, let's go to Shady Park. We'll have more fun there and we can go in the sprinklers and swing on those great swings there ..."

"Aghhhgrrr!!! NOOO!" Lina shrieked, so loudly that I felt my ears buzz. Then she whacked me in the face. Then she pinched my arm and kicked the shoes further away from herself. Most of the time I'm ready for this. I know that it's sometimes part of my life and I know what to do to make it better for everyone including Elsa. Acceptance, firm boundaries, and remaining centered are what ultimately console Lina, Elsa, and myself. But I wasn't there this time. I wanted Lina to change. Be different. Not scream. Not hit. Not make her little sister's life so challenging. Not make my life and her own so exhausting. So I yelled back.

"Put your shoes on, NOW!" I snapped. She immediately hit me. Then she threw her arms around me and wanted to be picked up. I picked her up just to hold her for a while, but she bit my shoulder hard, first on one side and then on the other.

Talking harshly to Lina never helps. It doesn't help her and it doesn't help Elsa and it helps me least of all. But I couldn't stop.

"Lina, you have no right to hit me! I know you're frustrated, but I'm not gonna let you whack me! Who ever hit you? We don't hit in this family," I said, feeling how my judgment tightened up my heart and my face and made me completely unavailable to myself or to Lina and painfully aware that everything I said and the hostility in my voice solved nothing.

Elsa knew. She wasn't even five years old yet but she knew that what I was saying didn't make any sense.

"Why do you tell her 'who ever hit you' when she can't help it?" she wanted to know.

"Because I'm tired of it," I said, feeling so low, having to explain my irrational behavior to someone who needed me to maintain the belief that Lina can't help that she sometimes hits and bites and screams and throws her shoes. Elsa, for the sake of her relationship with Lina, needs to know that I know that Lina doesn't have bad intentions, that it's not personal and it's not as bad as the world around us often thinks. She also, of course, needs to see that I'm setting firm boundaries for Lina. Just not in this way.

We walked toward the Riverside playground. Lina kept screaming. Throwing her shoes. Sitting down on the sidewalk. Whacking my arms. Pinching my legs. I held back. I pleaded. I got more pissed. I held her hand way too tightly. Nothing helped. The solution is not in Lina. My solution is within myself. But it was hidden this particular morning. As we got to the park, Lina swung for half a minute, then threw her shoes off and ran into the sprinklers and started pulling off her underwear. Then the dress. The water was three inches deep as usual in this park, with leaves and other debris clogging the drainage. It makes for a nice little kiddie pool. But for Lina, when she is in this kind of mood, it also makes for a nice little bathroom. Soon, with underwear and dress floating on the surface of the water, Lina bent down and peed. I was grateful it was just pee. Aware of the horrified looks of parents, park workers, and folks passing by, I chased Lina down, took her hand, and told her that we were going home. The walk home held more screaming and hitting and shoe throwing. I felt so desperate. As if there was nothing left inside to draw from. *Why* is not a good question to ask in these situations. I knew it would be much better to watch, do nothing, find stillness, than to act. But tears began to flow down my cheeks and panic gripped my stomach and I still had a big, noisy, neon blinking "WHY?" removing me from my source, preventing me from living with what is and moving from the "why" to the "how." But when I can't, life will. Half an hour later, Lina and Elsa and I were sitting by the kitchen table, smiling and chatting away as if nothing had happened, munching on lunch pancakes, Elsa's plain and Lina's drenched in casein-free butter.

Smiling and laughing at the many comical situations in our lives helps. Being in Lina's life, for almost everyone who spends more than a couple of hours at a time with her, is a very disorganizing experience. One time, we had a babysitter who froze into a full-blown panic attack, unable to do anything about Lina's escalating tantrum. By the time I decided to interrupt the play session to see if everything was okay, the babysitter was standing terrified in one corner of the room while Lina was throwing the CD player across the room. The rest of the room was in shambles. The babysitter's coffee was dumped on the floor as well and paintings were torn down from the walls and crushed against the floor. Lina had also broken two chairs in the short time before I came rushing in, and was in such an uncontrollable state that I brought her into the bedroom and held her down on the soft mattress until she slowly regained control.

Keeping one's cool is not just challenging because Lina is hyperactive and disorganized. The intensity of her disintegrated states often doesn't allow you enough time to maintain organized, rational behavior. Everything happens so fast. During one quite typical week, Sean lost his phone at the Bronx Zoo, Lina her shoes at school (it took us nearly half an hour and a lot of teachers searching for them before finding them under the thick mat in the sensory gym), two sweaters, also at school (and no, it's not because everyone is disorganized in her school; it's because they are around kids all day long who, like Lina, through no fault of their own, are equally disorganizing to their environment), I lost my phone, Tony his phone (in a cab) and his backpack, Emily (another babysitter) the keys to Tony's apartment . . . the list goes on.

In the middle of moving from one apartment to another right after we all came back to NYC from Rhode Island, Tony realized that his apartment keys were missing. He moved all his stuff out in the hallway, searching. But he had no success in finding the keys. So he thought to himself, "If I were Lina, where would I have put the keys?" The answer was as obvious to him as it would have been to me and anyone who spent a decent amount of time with our daughter. Out the window! Tony went to the only window that didn't have an air-conditioner in it, opened it, stuck his head out, and peered down. Three flights down, his keys were lying on a neighbor's air-conditioner. Tony smiled. He went down to the neighbor, explained his predicament, and picked up his keys.

At first, when babysitters started to get to places late when they were with Lina, lose keys to our houses and their own cell phones all over Manhattan, and bring Lina back home after spending time with her outdoors with only half of the clothing she was wearing when she left the house a couple of hours earlier, Tony and I had trouble keeping it in perspective. On the one hand the situation requires organized, efficient caregivers. On the other, phones, keys, strollers, backpacks, jackets, and hats will continue to get lost, by me and Tony as well as by our babysitters. It's just one more opportunity to learn acceptance. Of oneself and of others.

CHAPTER ELEVEN

Sisterhood

What follows was written by Elsa when she was six years old. I've included it within this book with her permission.

Good Job Lina!

Dedicated to Lina Lyons, for being my sister and friend. I'm proud of you!

Lina my sister has autism. But it was not always like that. When I was a baby Lina was a usual kid. In fact she was

*Really Gentle and she shared everything. But now it is hard
she screams "aaa"! and Kicks dramble dramble and laughs in
a funny way "ha ha ha" she is an 8-year old.*

*Because she has autism I learn a lot. But it is getting hard
explaining what autism is and because of that I have a
whole night with mama and a whole night with papa.
One dark night Lina had a Tantrum. She was screaming
"aa" she kicked on the couch dramble and laughed in a
funny way "ha ha ha." It was not just hard it Was really
super hard for me because It Was really super LOUD! And
it is hard because I can't Ask her to stop screaming she can't
Answer me! After the Tantrum was over it was time to
take a bath. Mom said "it is time to take a bath." I went
in the tub she jumped in splash the water went. Suddenly
Lina turned off the water she never did it before I said "did
you see that?" to mom "yes" said mom happily. I was super
proud of her.*

One warm, sunny fall afternoon, as I picked up five-year-old
Elsa from her kindergarten class, she hurried over to me and
melted into my arms. I could tell she was only one breath away
from tears.

"Mama, we were singing, 'Winter, Spring, Summer and Fall'
in school today ['All you have to do is call, and I'll be there, yes
I will. You've got a friend . . .'] and I wanted Lina, so badly!
But I didn't have anyone to talk to about it. Nobody listened,"
she said and choked on her last word, burying her head on my
shoulders. It was Wednesday, and Elsa's and my special day and
night. On Wednesdays, Sean played and worked with Lina until
Tony came back from work. Tony then had dinner with Lina
and kept her at his place while Elsa and I took the opportunity

to hang out just the two of us. Not infrequently, I would take Elsa on the back of my bike and go to the Swedish church on 5th Avenue and 48th Street. Eventually Elsa got too big for the bike's child seat and she would stand in front of me on the large scooter that fit both of us. For Elsa, the most enticing part of the Swedish church experience was the cinnamon buns. For me, it was the way the whole place smelled like Sweden as well as the kind of strong, black coffee that is so fundamental to the well-being of Swedes.

Wednesday is a day of carefree roaming around the city and the one day a week that I can devote wholeheartedly to Elsa. It invariably ends up with Elsa and me laughing and joking and making up silly stories way past bedtime and it helps us stay connected through the trials of our everyday life with Lina. I don't know which one of us needs and looks forward to these Wednesdays more. To me, it's the one solid day a week when I don't feel torn between the competing needs of my girls. To Elsa, it's the one day she can be just Elsa, and not the sister of a girl who never lets anyone predict what will happen next.

This particular afternoon, like many other Wednesdays, allowed Elsa the space to miss her sister. As we arrived outside our building later that day, Sean called to let me know that he'd decided to take Lina directly to Tony's house instead of stopping by my place first. I gave Elsa the phone so that she could say hi to Lina.

"Oh, Lina, I wanted you the whole day! Bye!"

Lina, impressed by and, as always, very sensitive to her little sister's expressions of love and affection, immediately responded, "Can I please have a home!" This was her way of saying that she wanted to be where Elsa was. Her way of saying, "Take me back to Elsa, I want her, too!"

Elsa processes her unusual life with a sister as unusual as Lina on multiple levels: in her pretend play and in her dreams, with Lina directly, and through her other relationships. Play acting, dancing, and singing are also important expressive relief for Elsa. Recognizing this resource in her, Tony and I enrolled Elsa in Lucy Moses summer camp and winter-break programs at the Kaufman Center on the Upper West Side. There she met Bess. Parents of kids with special needs can spot other kids with extra needs in seconds. Bess, with her charming and uncontrolled exuberance and almost nonexistent impulse control, was easily identifiable as a special kid. The first morning when I brought Elsa to Lucy Moses for the winter-break theater and music program I glanced at Bess and happily concluded to myself that the people here didn't just enroll perfectly well-behaved children. And I wasn't the only one who noticed. Elsa spotted Bess even before I did. Her reaction was interesting. She instantly felt both shy and full of admiration for this incessantly talkative nine-year-old girl with her short dark hair, bangs, and round, cherub-like physique. Elsa talked about Bess every day after the program, pondering with me about how to become Bess's friend. The last day of the camp, Elsa got sick, so she missed the recital that would have marked the end of her first camp at Lucy Moses. But much more upsetting to her than not being able to perform what she had practiced all week was the missed opportunity to make contact with Bess. Elsa was heartbroken.

Elsa, who makes friends with everyone in the world and surrounds herself with friends, both boys and girls, too numerous for me to keep track of had, I began to suspect, projected all her longings for closeness and explicit exchange with Lina onto Bess. She looked like someone feels after a bad breakup. As if the world had ceased to have color. The next day, as Elsa was listlessly walking to the playground, out of nowhere, as if in a dream, Bess came walking toward us on the sidewalk. She recognized Elsa and gave her a big hug. That was the beginning of an unlikely but beautiful friendship.

And I became close friends with Bess's babysitter, Nora. And Bess had a sibling. Jack, Bess's twin brother, was in a wheelchair and only able to communicate via a computer. We started to arrange playdates with everyone—Lina, Jack, Elsa, Bess, Nora, and I—on Saturdays. These were interesting events, to put it mildly, including one occasion when Bess rearranged my entire closet, emptied its contents, and spread it all out on the floor in the playroom. As Bess often does, she retrospectively realized that this may not have been Elsa's mom's favorite game. But whatever drama or intrigue we encountered on these get-togethers, they involved way more laughing than crying, much more acceptance than judgment, and a lot of good times and good lunches for all six of us.

In September of 2009 Elsa had started prekindergarten. A few months into that fall, her teacher noticed that Elsa had some discomfort with her socks and that clothing with seams bothered her. Elsa had shown some mild sensory avoidant behavior when we had lived in Newport, too, and I had decided to watch it for a while and, if it didn't improve, evaluate her with an occupational therapist. That summer, exposed to weather and wind, sand and water, soil and mud, and anything else we could find in the parks around the city, she became bolder. But when facing the stressors of a new school and new friends, some of that sensory discomfort returned. Elsa's teacher had also noticed that Elsa easily became afraid of dramatic content in books, and that she sometimes became very upset and scared when the boys in her class became pretend warriors and dragons and even firefighters.

I took her to Jan Drucker, the psychology professor at Sarah Lawrence who had been my teacher when I got my masters in child development there in the early nineties. I had never forgotten her unique understanding of children. And I figured, if there is one person you want to know as much as possible about before letting your child meet them, it's your little one's therapist. So the thought of Jan Drucker meeting with Elsa made me happy. She has a gift. It was as if someone had given her magic 3-D glasses that gave her insights into the world and the dynamics of children. I re-experienced myself as a student in her classes. And I brought everything I had learned from this unusually intelligent woman to the Karen Horney Clinic where I did my fieldwork and later stayed on to work. The clinic focused on kids with social and emotional trauma. And while Elsa's experience was very different from the kids at Karen Horney, Elsa had certainly been through so much more than most kids her age ever had to deal with. For the last couple of years, she had seen her sister go from verbal and calm to losing most of her vocabulary, and becoming incontinent and desperately sensory-seeking which included the biting and the pouring and the ripping and the running and jumping and screaming and not sleeping that affected Elsa at least as much as it did me and Tony. She also experienced my mother's death, which made her afraid of me dying, the end of her parents' marriage, multiple moves, the loss of close friends. I wanted to give her a chance now, rather than her having to do it twenty years from now, to process the situations in her life that become so overwhelming.

Elsa jumped on the opportunity. Jan Drucker became "The Lady" and Elsa's steps always became faster and more eager when on the way to her office. She played in there as if her life depended on it. She marched in with the focus of a tiger that, hungry for weeks, had just spotted a nearby gazelle. She composed her sessions as if she had a pre-set schedule to adhere to and Jan reported that, like clockwork, wherever she left off, down to the very detail, she picked up the next session. While Elsa's therapy sessions are her own, private and sacred, her need to process the experience of her sister's challenges and everyone's reactions, including her own, to such challenges, became abundantly clear. She sometimes invited me into her sessions, and I saw my own helplessness and frustration in trying to make home life manageable, from the eyes of my four-and-a-half-year-old girl. But I also saw how having this wise outsider's support in processing a challenging childhood helped Elsa grow more bold, more expressive, less shy of sensory input, and increasingly comfortable with all the different situations in her life, including relating to Lina. During this time Elsa's unusual flair for dramatic expression surfaced with even more gusto. I welcomed it, knowing that she was trying to set things straight, going from adjusting to Lina to making her own presence increasingly noticeable. One day, Elsa was upset about a couple of drawings I had made of Pippi Longstocking. The last straw for Elsa was the fact that I had put blue in the middle of Pippi's dress and that the color had covered the buttons. Elsa started to cry out loud and as she calmed down slightly to put words on her despair, she said, "This is so terrible! My heart cannot exist anymore!"

Her increasingly liberated dramatic expression took many forms. One day during this same period, Elsa and I were playing Winnie the Pooh and Piglet. We were pretending to sleep.

Elsa: "Wake up! I have so much energy. I can feel my bones struggling!"

Elsa's fear of me dying, in the context of her grandmother's death, also became more explicit during this time. One night, Elsa and I were talking about dying.

Elsa: "I'm gonna have to die when you die, cause I love you."

Back at school after a long summer the following year, with hours and hours of outdoor time, Elsa's sensory processing issues were no longer noticeable. Her mid-semester kindergarten evaluation described "joy of learning" and "excitement for school" and how "each day she arrived with a smile on her face and a warm greeting for her classmates and teachers." I wept as I read that Elsa is "patient, sensitive, and caring ... thoughtful and well liked by her peers" and "a wonderful member of the classroom community." It was the first time since Lina was three and a half years old that I had taken part in an evaluation of one of my children in which everything was just fine and no one was concerned about any aspect of my child's development. Elsa had moved from fear to acceptance, welcoming her sister's neurological unpredictability with open, loving arms, getting her own life back on track, finding emotional relief and creative expression in her drawings, singing, dancing, and storytelling, and developing an empathetic sensibility well beyond her years. With such accomplishments came a lot of talking directly about what was going on with Lina. At one point, Elsa had a conversation with Tony about autism.

Elsa: Lina has autism.

Tony: What does autism mean to you?

Elsa: Well, it means that Lina can't eat certain things, and she can't really talk . . . and, Lina can't stop thinking about all the things she wants.

Instinctively, Elsa knows how to reach Lina. She recognizes every little subtlety and knows exactly when to expand on the interaction between them. When Lina sits down to cut up magazines on the floor in my office next to the kitchen, where we spend a lot of our time when we are not in the playroom, Elsa sits down next to her, she also with scissors. Then she starts commenting on the pictures and Lina starts listening. It's so much easier and more compelling for Lina to imitate Elsa than any of the adults in her life. Soon, Lina makes her own brief but spontaneous comments on some of the pictures in the magazines and joint attention is established without anyone's calculations and planning.

At the dinner table, we often discuss food, which is the one subject that comes naturally to Lina. "Can I please have a scone," Lina will say. Elsa, who also likes scones, joins in and says she wants that, too. Then we think together about when would be a good time to make scones, tomorrow morning or on Sunday morning when we have more time. Music is another point of connection. Lina is the obvious DJ and then there is dancing and singing and discussions together about the music. Both Elsa and I love Lina's music choices, which makes the whole experience very gratifying to Lina. It is so clear that whenever she actually gets involved in a conversation or an activity, she loves to be part of things. And Elsa is so happy whenever it seems as if she is actually having a conversation or some other kind of interaction with Lina.

In the winter of 2011, Lina was becoming increasingly fascinated with her little sister. At the dinner table, she often stopped eating and leaned over toward Elsa's chair and just watched her, with her face half an inch away from Elsa's. Sometimes Elsa loved the attention, sometimes she didn't. If Elsa moved to a different chair to get some space, Lina seemed aware of the rejection, and sometimes made a little protest shout, to make sure we all knew she would rather have Elsa back next to her. On Tuesday evenings, when Elsa has her Papa night, Lina has the bathtub all to herself. But now Lina started to say, "Can I please have a Elsa!" whenever she registered that Elsa hadn't shown up in the bathtub with her. By asking for Elsa whenever she wasn't around, Lina seemed to be saying that her world was better with her sister in it. Her little sister loves her and accepts her in an effortless, genuine way that few others can. At the same time, Elsa has a vision for Lina. She is looking forward to the day they can have secrets together and play Ariel and Snow White games together. One day, Elsa was hanging out at Tony's publishing office with one of his editors, Jennifer McCartney. After their meeting, Jennifer described how Elsa had drawn a picture of a woman, a girl, and a mermaid. She pointed and said: "This is me, this is the mom, and this is the older sister. She is a mermaid. She is trapped in her body but one day she'll be free."

CHAPTER TWELVE

Fear of Breakdown

L ike Elsa, I believe there will be a day when Lina will be free. I cannot let myself look into the future and see Lina's challenges intensifying. I just can't do it. It has to get better. I will understand her more. She will be able to show me more. We will find something that will help her feel less anxious, happier, and more connected and fulfilled. In my darkest moments, my biggest fear is that I won't last until that day comes. Some weeks and months are more challenging than others. The winter and early spring of 2011 was one such time.

Lina had spent weeks screaming in almost every situation—at the dinner table, in the store, on the street, and in the playground.

One such day, I took Lina to our favorite grocery store, Fairway, to get the olives that she loves so much, some eggs, and organic strawberries. We got to the cashier when Lina started up. Her sudden and unexpected shrieks made everyone, the thirty cashiers, security staff, and managers, the delivery people, and the customers crowding in long checkout lines, freeze. The huge store suddenly got very quiet.

"Can I please have olives!! AAAGGHHRR!!"

I kneeled down and explained in a calm voice to Lina that she would get them as soon as we got home. It made no impression on her.

"CAN I PLEASE HAVE A OLIVES!!! AAAGGHRRRRRRIIII!"

"She can't help it, no impulse control," I told the genuinely concerned, on the brink of terrified, cashier. She looked panicky. Lina still screamed.

"Don't worry, she'll be okay," I smiled encouragingly while pressing Lina's head against my stomach to give her the sensory support she needs in these out-of-control moments. I paid, threw the food in bags, and took Lina's hand. I tried to move slowly and calmly to counteract Lina's escalating anxiety. Lina kept screaming. I kept walking, trying to hold her hand as gently as I could while still getting us out and home as soon as humanly possible. Outside, Lina kicked the bags and screamed even louder. I sat down in front of her, trying to speak to her in the most simple terms that maybe she could still hear while her arms were flailing and her thoughts racing and her own screams taking her to a place where it was so hard to reach her. Somehow we managed to cross the street. Lina kept kicking the bags and wailing and hit me in the face three times in a row before I could even catch her arms to contain her. A long row of passersby, the store's security guards, and customers were lined up by the corner on the other side of the street, watching and talking about what they had just seen, wondering what I would do next. As in most cases, I did nothing other than try to keep myself and Lina safe, talking to her softly, waiting it out. Lina, on the other hand, jumped up and ran over to a café that's on our street, pulled the flowers and soil from the little flower boxes outside the café, and threw them on the ground. The café owner, a tall, now indignant woman came out.

"What's going on?" she asked in a loud, authoritarian voice that demanded to know. I looked at her and estimated that she and I, as well as Lina, would benefit from a decision to keep quiet at this time. I quickly swiped up the flower and as much soil as I could catch in one sweep, and planted it back in the flower box. Then I took Lina's hand, grabbed our grocery bags, and started to walk home. Lina screamed all the way to our building. At home, as she was munching quietly on the black and green olives by the kitchen table, familiar tears rolled down my cheeks.

A couple of peaceful minutes went by, with Lina munching on the olives, seeming okay, smiling at me, saying, "I want to pick berries. Can I please pick berries?" I understood it as conversational, dreaming about picking berries, saying something that comes easily for her, expressing an idea of something that gives her a good feeling. She talks about picking berries all year round. I engaged her, trying to help her elaborate and build on it, placing it in time, going back to retrieve memories of picking berries, using something that motivates Lina to expand our exchange. At some point, Lina became restless again. Now she wanted to throw the rest of the olives out. She wanted other things to eat.

She wanted me to fry an egg for her and as soon as I did, without tasting it, she wanted to throw it out. Then she wanted cupcakes, fresh figs, and gingersnap cookies. My response was, "We don't have that today, Lina, but if you want . . ."

"NO!!" she screamed back before I had finished the sentence and jumped up and down, threw a left hook into my stomach, dumped the olives all over the kitchen floor, ran out of the kitchen, threw down the coat hanger, and rushed over to Elsa's room and tried to turn over the bookshelves that are the divider between Elsa's room and the living room while at the same time grabbing a bag of coins and flinging them all over the living room. Everything was accompanied by the kind of screaming sounds that make most people want to call an ambulance. Not me. I knew that a few seconds later my daughter's face might break out in a warm, relaxed smile. Until the next outburst. All I knew was that I didn't know when the next crisis would hit. Whenever Lina gets to this place, I try to remind both her and myself that she is trying to come to terms with whatever is going on in her system. That she is doing the best she can with whatever she has at that moment. Maybe the intensity of her tantrum is the extent to which she wants to figure out her world. Maybe she is screaming because she is in some kind of pain that we haven't yet been able to alleviate.

We were in the playground and Lina was climbing on a wooden bridge that connected two slides. As she was standing in the middle of the bridge, she suddenly started to scream and jump up and down in frustration. A little girl stood in the sand right under the bridge, following Lina's every move.

"She doesn't mean anything by it," I reassured her. The girl looked at me and nodded. Lina screamed louder. The girl kept looking right at her, not moving an inch from where she was standing right under Lina.

"It's not as bad as it sounds," I added with a smile.

"I know."

"You know?"

The girl nodded. This one clearly didn't need my explanations. I smiled. It doesn't matter if it comes from a little preschool kid or a wise old lady or someone in between. Acceptance and understanding are the blessings that get us through the day no matter what happens.

Every day during this period held new challenges. Lina seemed to spend more and more time being in a completely disintegrated state. Her movements became increasingly jerky and less purposeful. The threshold between being calm and starting to scream, roll around on the ground, kick her shoes off, and hit whoever was with her wherever she could, seemed lower and lower until it became difficult even to distinguish the threshold. I felt a kind of tiredness inside that I had never felt before. Something that couldn't give anymore and couldn't take anymore. Something inside that just wanted to scream right out in space, to make everything that was, stop. One Sunday night after the girls had spent the afternoon and evening at Tony's place, Lina sat down on a chair for a few seconds. I could tell she was not happy. Tony had told me that she hadn't wanted to get out of the cab. She loves riding in cars and this car ride only lasted the seven blocks that separated my house from Tony's. She had been screaming and kicking, trying to stay in the car, until Tony simply had to lift her out of there and bring her inside. Tony hurried off, having left his cell phone in the cab in the midst of all the commotion. Now, back home, Lina jumped up and started to scream, threw down the coat hanger, which broke, then ran over to the bookshelf and started to throw books on the floor in Elsa's room.

"No, Lina! I'm *not* gonna let you destroy our whole house!" I yelled, ending up so far away from who I wanted to be that I wanted to yell even louder. I wanted to yell at myself for yelling. I wanted to throw ten coat hangers on the floor to express my own frustration about not being who I felt I needed to be. But before I could think one more sad, desperate thought, Elsa expressed her side of the story.

"I am so tired!" she cried and disappeared into the playroom, curling up on the couch. "I can't do it anymore, I'm so tired of the screaming!" she sobbed.

I dropped everything and followed Elsa into the playroom.

"I know, my love, I'm so sorry," I said, feeling the despair of the inconsolable conflict between the needs of my two children. As I was standing there, looking at Elsa crying about the mayhem she so often was forced to experience right at bedtime, Lina started to throw books and rip the pages in the other room. "Wait, I'll be right back."

In Elsa's room, Lina was laughing, grabbing the books and slugging them across the room. There were books everywhere, some ripped, some still intact.

"Stop it, Lina!" was the only thing I could think of saying before I realized that I was better off giving both Lina and myself some more space before getting into more interactions with her. I went back to the playroom.

"How are you, baby?" I ask Elsa, who now had closed her eyes, doing what she could to exclude the parts of her daily life that had become too much for her.

"Okay."

"No, you are not okay. You don't have to say that you're okay when you're not!"

She started sobbing. "I'm so tired of the screaming! I just want to be able to sleep!"

"I'm so sorry, I understand. Of course you do. Is there anything else you want to tell me?"

"I wanted to give you a hug but you were just running from room to room trying to stop Lina!"

"Baby, I understand, but you don't have to fix this. You don't have to comfort me. I should comfort you. I'm your mama."

I sat on the couch quietly for a moment, holding Elsa's hand. Then asked her:

"Do you want to tell me more about what you're feeling?"

"No, well, one more thing. It's hard for me because when I get here I'm so tired and then the screaming starts and I just want to be able to sleep."

"I'm so sorry, baby. I'll try to figure it out. Thank you for telling me about what it is like for you."

The evening ended like most evenings did during this period, before I came up with the very good idea of putting a hammock in the playroom. Elsa fell asleep on the couch holding my hand while Lina was curled up in my lap, facing me on the large exercise ball, bouncing to the rhythms of Nina Simone, Stevie Wonder, Akon.

As we were sitting there, Lina looked at me and suddenly said:

"I'm not sorry."

It was as if she had thought about it and wanted to make sure I understood that she cannot help it and to remind me not to get mad at her.

"I know. That's okay, Lina. I know you're doing the best you can. We're both doing the best we can."

But Lina had more she wanted to tell me.

"I'm sorry for getting mad."

"Lina, thank you for telling me. I understand. You don't mean it. And I'm sorry, too. I love you."

Later, Tony called to let me know he was coming to bring an antibacterial cream that Elsa needed. I told him the truth as I thought he deserved a fair warning, should I not make it.

"Tony, I'm not sure how long I'm going to be able to do this. Just so you know, I'm contemplating renting a car and driving to a different life. And you should know, I'm not kidding."

Somehow, the evening ended with Tony and me sitting around eating ice cream, laughing about our failed marriage, Lina's latest pranks, and our own imperfect ways of dealing with them.

The next morning, Lina had not spent more than five minutes in the kitchen before getting disregulated and was soon screaming at the top of her lungs, anxious to throw her just-finished fried egg in the garbage and looking around for more things to throw, somewhere. The French press coffeepot came into her view and before anyone had blinked, coffee was everywhere— on the walls, inside the pots-and-pans cabinet, dripping from the kitchen counter, covering most of the floor. I calmly asked Lina to go sit on the couch and lifted Elsa from her chair onto the couch as well. I started cleaning up. Somehow, the three of us eventually got out of the house. With Elsa having a day off from school, I decided to bring her with me to drop Lina off at school. Lina screamed most of the way there, asking for rice cakes, throwing them on the ground, requesting another one. In her never-ending quest for sugar, Lina spotted a neon green piece of candy on the ground and quickly put it in her mouth. But in the end, most of this green stuff came out. The stickiness on Lina's hand helped solidify my grip on her and made it harder for her to suddenly pull out of my hand and chase down some other colorful treasure on the sidewalk. You lose some and win some, I smiled to myself. Those are the little details that will make a mother of a sensory-seeking child smile. After we dropped Lina off, with added screams and kicking, an hour and a half late to school, I walked with Elsa into a café, the first one I could find, and just sank into the chair opposite my daughter, her chattering fading to the background. I just stared off into the distance, wondering what would happen to us. It felt as if I had taken myself and my daughter on a path that suddenly ended in front of a steep and bottomless pit. I had never been so deeply tired.

On another afternoon, Elsa walked into a construction pole after, without my knowing it, she tried to figure out if she could walk down the street to our building with her eyes closed. Blood was gushing from her nose and as soon as we came inside, Lina matched Elsa's tears with her own high-pitched screams and accompanying right hooks into my belly. She should have been a boxer. There was so much force in that hit that I had to gasp for air. I know she just wanted my attention and my help to regulate herself. But Elsa was sobbing on the couch so I asked Sean to take Lina into the playroom while I wiped the blood off my other daughter's face. Sean did, but Lina ran out of the room before Sean had the chance to stop her and before I had the chance to blink, Lina had bit right into my right breast. There was a British psychoanalyst, Melanie Klein, who came up with theories about how young children, in the separation-individuation process, in their minds attack their mothers' breasts. In my mind, looking down at the extra circle around the areola on my breast, I wondered if Melanie Klein ever had experienced her own theories as concretely and tangibly as this. There was much more to this day, but somehow the three of us ended up getting through it and falling asleep that night.

But it was the next night that Lina had one of the worst tantrums that I have seen. I had been with Elsa and was picking up Lina, who had been with Sean at Tony's place. As always on Tuesdays, Lina and I were going to have our special evening as Elsa was to stay with Tony. As Lina was leaving, she completely fell apart, screaming and rolling around on the ground, hitting and biting. She had wanted the cereal that was in Tony's place, did not want to leave, and threw herself on the ground outside Tony's building. The doorman tried to offer some water.

"No thanks, she is not able to drink right now." Another lady stopped with her dog and asked if there was anything she could do.

"No, thank you. It's okay."

The doorman moved closer, and asked, "Where is Sean?"

"Listen, Sean went home, I'm here, she'll be fine. Is there anything else you want to say to me, anything helpful or otherwise? As you can see I'm kind of busy," I snapped, while trying to keep Lina's head from banging into the protruding air-conditioner and the hard ground. Another lady from the building walked up with a glass of water. *What's up with the water? Do they really think she is able to focus on drinking water right now?* I asked myself, amazed and pissed off at how help-less we all are in the face of someone falling apart. Before I had a chance to project any of my own despair explicitly on someone else, Lina knocked the water glass out of the lady's hand, sending the glass, the water, and the ice cubes flying through the air. I shrugged my shoulders and said, "Thanks, though." Somehow, we got home. We spent hours in the kitchen. Lina was standing by the kitchen counter, eating cabbage salad, which she occasionally spiced up with Nigerian cayenne pepper. As she was standing there, gradually calming down from the massive emotional and neurological tornado she had just been in the midst of, she suddenly said:

"Go to the spirit world."

It was a good idea. I think it was her way of saying, *We need help, beyond this material world. In the spiritual world we can find relief.* The next day, after more shrieking, thrown bananas, rolling around on the sidewalk, jumping up and down in sheer frustration, as if she was about to crawl out of her own skin, I went home and called my best friend.

"Gabriella, something isn't holding together inside. I'm afraid of what will happen. It is as if Lina has slipped into a permanently disregulated state. She is making less and less sense. It is as if her world is becoming more and more incoherent and overwhelming. I feel so helpless and angry," I sobbed into the phone, experi-encing a kind of surreal feeling of drifting off of my own center. "Can you help me? Could you do something or send something to get us through the day?" My wise shaman friend did not say very much. But she did exactly what I had asked her to do.

That day was different from any day we had experienced for months. Lina didn't scream once. She whimpered a few times over the course of the afternoon, but overall she was happier and more comfortable, smiley, and affectionate than I had seen her for a long time. Dinner proceeded without a single scream. No food was thrown on the floor and Lina didn't try to tilt over the table or anything else a single time. Elsa and I were in shock. Why is it always at one's breaking point that mercy shows up? I felt grateful and confused. But after this day, little by little, things improved. It seemed as if the edge of her despair had somehow fallen off.

In *The Way of the Shaman*, Michael Harner describes how "the shaman shares his special powers and convinces his patients, on a deep level of consciousness, that another human is willing to offer up his own self to help them" (1990, p. xvii). When nothing else works, and Lina herself tells me that she wants to "go to the spirit world," I will listen.

It's not just Lina. Most of us do it. When life takes us to places where we see no way out, where everything on the outside seems closed, overwhelming, and impossible, we look for answers on the inside and in the space beyond our physical life. I think it is instinct. I think it is meant to be that way. In fact, I think that is one of the benefits of very challenging times. If we let it, it can soften us and bring us closer to the very best part of ourselves and our humanity. The Tibetan Buddhist Pema Chodron, in *When Things Fall Apart* (1997, p. 15–16), writes:

> When we reach our limit, if we aspire to know that place
> fully—which is to say that we aspire to neither indulge nor
> repress—a harness in us will dissolve. We will be softened
> by the sheer force of whatever energy arises—the energy of
> anger, the energy of disappointment, the energy of fear. When

it's not solidified in one direction or another, the very energy pierces us to the heart, and it opens us. This is the discovery of egolessness. It's when all our usual schemes fall apart. Reaching our limit is like finding a doorway to sanity and the unconditional goodness of humanity, rather than meeting an obstacle or punishment.

Lina responds profoundly to anyone who gets to this point and, instead of shutting down and withdrawing, or overreacting and lashing out, stays present, vulnerable, and honest, right there with her. Like the day when everything fell apart for her and she kicked, screamed, punched me in the face, threw things, ran around the apartment like a wild animal, and finally, both of us exhausted, calmed down and sank down on the couch. Then she suddenly stood up and walked quickly back and forth between the kitchen and my office, preparing to say something.

"I'm lost. You cannot find her!"

I look at her. I knew this was communication directly from her heart.

"I know, Lina. You are right. I can see that you are lost."

"Say, I'm lost, you CANNOT find her," she said again with added intensity.

"Lina, I know that is true. I cannot find her. I cannot do it alone. I need your help."

Lina was quiet for a moment, but very still and very present. Then she looked at me and said:

"Have to wait."

"Okay, Lina, I'll wait. I'll wait for when you're ready."

Lina and I were hanging out in the playroom one day, she in the hammock, me on the mat next to her. Lina was in a splendid mood. I pushed her high in the hammock and caught her on the down turn. Unable to contain her excitement and express her wish to keep playing in words, she came swinging toward me at full speed, widely grinning, and kicked me with all her might in the side of my head. With sign language, words, and facial expression, I tried to explain to my delightedly giggling girl that kicking wasn't the same as playing. Maintaining her big, beautiful, irresistible smile that somehow always strikes me as larger than life, she leaned forward and responded:

"Good to see you, too!"

CHAPTER THIRTEEN

Trial and Error: Various Alternative Methods of Treatment

For parents of children with special needs, there will never be a time when one can sit down and say: we know what works and what doesn't work and we're doing everything we can to help our son or daughter. There are always more evaluations to be done, new diets to try, other treatment approaches that were not right for one's child a year ago but might be now. There are medicines and supplements to try out and insurance issues to clarify. I ask myself on an ongoing basis, how should I most effectively work with Lina? Who, at any given point, should be involved in Lina's care? How many transitions each day, from one person to the next, from one setting to another, is reasonable to expect Lina to handle? What biomedical supplements should she take and how much? Which doctors should be involved in her care? When will it benefit Lina to come to a relative's birthday party or some other social event and when will it be torture for her, given her inclination for sensory overload, all the things she cannot eat, and all the things she cannot do at such events?

One beautiful, sunny October afternoon, Tony and I tried to figure out whether we should bring Lina to his mother's birthday party. The fact that Lina's antiviral diet now allowed for pasta became the decisive factor for us this time. "Let's try to bring her this time and then we'll talk about how it went later," I suggested. Everyone else had already taken a seat in Tony's parents' apartment when Lina arrived. She quietly sat down next to me on the couch. I reminded her that it was Grandma's birthday and at that Lina looked over at Grandma and, with everyone's eyes on her, spontaneously started to sing, "Happy birthday to you! Happy birthday to you! Happy birthday to Grandmaaaa, happy birthday to you!" It was beautiful and the rest of that party went on in the same cooperative, smiley, peaceful manner. Over the course of the meal, Lina now and then walked over to Grandma, gave her a kiss, checked out the table in front of her for any interesting foods she might lay her hands on, smiled warmly at Grandma, and walked back to her own spot on the couch next to me. By the end of the meal, Tony and I, blown away by our little queen's exceptional behavior, were ready to take her out of special school and stop attending any further IEP meetings. And now, Lina was definitely coming to the next family gathering.

During the same fall of 2010, Tony and I were also considering the following: Should we introduce a more behavioral approach at this point to complement the DIR, floor-time methodology that Lina received in school? Should we add more hours in the playroom again? While we still tried to spend as much focused time in the playroom as possible on both weekdays and weekends, with Lina in school Monday through Friday, she spent much more time in the classroom than in the playroom. We wondered if she would benefit from a school with a little more structure than what Rebecca School offered. That year, the board of education recommended a school downtown in Battery Park, and we wondered if that might be an option for Lina.

One ongoing issue that we were facing continually at Rebecca School was the high turnover of staff. Hiring a lot of young, energetic people presumably at low salaries had its down- and upsides. What they lacked in experience, they made up for with enthusiasm. They were interested and motivated to learn but soon moved on to better-paying jobs. Trying to get a sense of all our options, I went to visit the school that the board of education had offered. The speech therapist, occupational therapist, and teachers seemed fine. Their attitude seemed almost as relational and personable as the teachers at Lina's current school. But there was no large sensory equipment in the classroom; no bouncy things that would help Lina calm down when she was falling apart. And they had no sensory gym. I envisioned my daughter losing all she had gained through our work in the playroom and at Rebecca School and disintegrating in the face of so many additional transitions and declined the placement, signing Lina up for another year at Rebecca School. Tony and I hoped that the board of education would continue to reimburse us for the Rebecca School tuition, gradually climbing closer to a yearly $100,000.

Antiviral Medication

During this time, Tony and I were also considering a trial of anti-viral medicine for Lina. After a month of Lina taking carnosine, under the advice of Dr. Lynch, he also agreed to put her on an antiviral medication. Since Lina had shown her first autism symp-toms in the context of her second MMR shot and subsequent Epstein-Barr virus exposure when she was three and a half years old, I had always thought it would make sense to try an antiviral. After preparing carefully with anti-yeast treatments including giving Lina a nasty-tasting anti-yeast powder, Nystatin, and adding more probiotic remedies to Lina's twice-daily medication cocktails, Dr. Lynch prescribed the strong antiviral medication called Valtrex. While the differences between hope and objective evaluation of various treatments are very difficult for a parent of a child with autism, Valtrex seemed promising. With no one other than me and Tony knowing about the new medication, reports by others in Lina's life pointed toward improved social related-ness, shorter and less intense tantrums, more cooperative behavior, and a little bit more deliberate language. In his ongoing progress notes on playroom sessions and outdoor time with Lina, Sean noted much less screaming in transitions, with more collabora-tion and responsiveness in the playroom. Sean also noticed how Lina seemed more interested in other kids. When Tony's and my friends Tad and Susan and their twelve-year-old son Christopher were over for dinner at Tony's house, Sean reported, Lina kept following Christopher around, jumping on the bouncing ball with him and watching him closely wherever he went.

In the playroom, with both Sean and me, Lina began to actively request reading books, and sometimes even initiated redoing the puzzle she had just completed. She sang songs together with us as opposed to just filling in the words when we stopped singing to encourage her to get involved. She threw a ball thirty times back and forth, while counting and maintaining eye contact, and even with a smile on her face. I wasn't sure if this was Valtrex or just her general development, but I was sure I would continue this trial for another couple of months just as Dr. Lynch had recommended for as long as there seemed to be a likely correlation. These are the life lessons autism teaches. If one is a control freak or is a perfectionist, one runs straight into a wall. Autism teaches patience. Acceptance. Endurance. Creativity. Independent thinking. Letting go of the need for environmental approval. It's trial and error. It's about trying to stay open to multiple solutions. Maybe Valtrex was making Lina feel better. Maybe it wasn't. For as long as it seemed like a possibility, I kept crushing those little blue pills each morning and night and mixing them into her "jam treat," a concoction that was a twice-daily routine to disguise Valtrex and a number of other supplements. It involved a spoonful of sugar-free jam, further inspired by a few drops of the sweetener Stevia, dusted with a layer of cinnamon, and uplifted by a little fresh lemon juice.

Integrating ABA with a Relational Approach—Round One: Giving it a Try

In the spirit of scrolling down the list of things Tony and I agreed to try in order to help Lina as efficiently as we could, I contacted Jennifer Clark, who had written a PhD dissertation on the subject of integrating ABA (applied behavioral analysis) and DIR (developmental, individual-difference, relationship-based). Just as I don't like to give my child strong medications that involve multiple potential side effects, I don't much like ABA. But this effort to help Lina is no longer about what I like. It's not even necessarily always about what Lina likes. It's kind of a combination of what Lina needs and wants. Lina used to be extremely self-directed. Gradually, she became a little less so and a little bit more like a partner to whomever she was working with. Maybe now, I thought, it was time to impose more of our vision of behavior on this little freedom-hungry fairy. Maybe it would be okay now to introduce a little bit of behavior modification. I was willing to try it out. Tony was eager.

I knew I needed help with this. When I was in my twenties, I had worked as an ABA therapist with a little girl who had autism. I loved working with her, but instead of feeling that the rigid exercises we plowed through and checked off were the most important part of our work together, I had the intuitive understanding that our relationship survived that part, and that somehow this little wonderful girl knew it, too. One afternoon, this girl, who never said anything spontaneously, and very rarely showed or expressed emotion, came up to me, hugged me, and said, "I love you, Helena!" As I bent down and held this little girl in my arms, I looked up at her mother's bewildered face. Pain and excitement. Loss and gain. Heartbreak and joy. It was all in her face.

"I think you will hear it soon," I said to her. "I think it was meant for you."

But one night, all the ABA therapists were gathering for a session to help our little friend with toilet training. The invasiveness of us all being there in the living room, cheering on the crying, scared girl to encourage her to approach the potty placed in the middle of the room, became too much for me. I told her father as we were driving to the train station to drop me off, "I don't believe in this." Later he called me.

"Helena, you understand why I called you, eh?"

"Tell me anyway."

"You don't believe in this. . . . We can't let you work with us anymore. You have a nice relationship with our daughter and we appreciate what you've done for us but we need people who are 100 percent with the program."

And now, twenty years later, it was my turn. I called Jennifer Clark. We met, discussed Lina, and agreed that she would help me create a book for Lina. It involved matching, working on her name, and social questions for the first round. The first time I introduced it to Lina was a complete disaster and we both ended up in tears after Lina tore up the book with social questions and pictures that I had spent the evening before making up. Eventually, things got a little easier. I encouraged Sean and Stephanie (another babysitter who was with us at the time) to try to introduce more structure in the sessions, and work more intensively on numbers, her name, colors, spatial relationships, etc. And I began to try out the idea of imposing our reality and vision and expectations on Lina. "You sit by the table through these exercises and then we'll bounce." "You'll help me build and count the blocks of this tower and then we'll listen to a song." "You'll match these shapes and tell me the colors and then we'll have a snack." It's all a matter of focus. It all sounds benign. But Lina wasn't ready. She started to mix up the colors, answer out of context, zone out, and, with a despair and rawness I have never seen in her, scream and lose control and show aggression in a way that I hadn't experienced since that spring three years ago in Rhode Island, when Lina's difficulties started. Lina had outbursts at school, too. Her despair and the level of complete disintegration made even her teacher, Jill, lose her cool and break down crying. On our way to school one of those mornings, an icy, cold morning, Lina again started screaming suddenly. She kicked off her boots and refused to put them back on. I looked at her feet and striped socks unprotected on the wet, icy sidewalk. I wanted to force her to stop doing things that hurt her. I wanted to pretend that I was in control and make her do what I wanted. But deep inside, I knew she was trying to tell me something. I took her hand in one hand and her boots in the other and went to a little dry spot under a door entrance. I found a soft, open, sad space inside and decided not to cover it up.

"Lina, please, my love, I'm asking you, let me help you put the boots on. It's so cold." Tears dripped down my cheeks as I looked at my little girl, making her statement, confused about why suddenly her world involved so many people trying to manipulate her into doing things instead of being with her. She looked at me for a few seconds, leaned forward, and kissed me on my mouth. Then she helped me put her boots on, took my hand, and walked briskly with me to school, softly singing.

That same morning, Elisabeth, Lina's special DIR therapist at Rebecca, whom Lina loves so much and who is completely in love with Lina and hugs me as if I have given her a million-dollar lotto ticket every time I see her in the hallways of Rebecca School, brought me into an empty room after drop-off, closed the door, and asked me, "What's going on? Lina has been so disregulated lately!"

I thought about it. I thought about Lina. I listened to my heart. And I took a step back. I don't want to impose my world on Lina. I want to make it attractive enough for her to want to be in it. And I want to keep learning about hers. So I talked to Tony, Sean, and everyone else involved in Lina's life about taking a step back, to again prioritize their engagement with Lina and elicit learning in the situations that interest Lina naturally. I decided to trust that all the rest would come in time. It was as if a switch in Lina's brain went off. Lina, who had been so out of it for the past two weeks, screaming and kicking as if she knew her own integrity was at stake, began to smile again. Her screaming subsided. Her speech became more coherent. Her interactions more deliberate. The night after I had told Sean to go back to plan A, he came back to the house, glowing. He and Lina had been in Central Park and on the way home, Lina kept saying, "We're going to Mama's house," and pulling his arm.

"I know, Lina, that's what we're doing!" But Lina kept pulling his arm in protest and pointing out that they were going to "Mama's house." Then Sean realized he had walked down 75th Street instead of 74th, and Lina had noticed and tried to redirect him! So we decided to hold off with the behavioral approach for a couple of months, to see if Lina would get to a place where she was more ready for it.

Let's just say that to have someone like Sean around, who can implement new plans, new trials, new approaches quicker than I can think them out, is in itself a miracle. Every day that he is around, he comes into the house with a friendly smile, the most cheerful and energetic approach, exuding willingness and ability to do whatever is necessary. Thinking and working and constantly evaluating and trying out different strategies in helping Lina at all the different phases of her life is much more workable with this unusual twenty-six-year-old from Wisconsin around.

Equine Assisted Therapy—A Failed Attempt

The next trial was to get Lina back into horseback riding. With Lina still fitting into the child seat at the back of my bicycle, we went to a city stable in Hell's Kitchen, which is an area west of midtown that's less crowded and that hosts a few stables, one of which offers riding to special-needs children. As soon as I lifted Lina out of the bike seat, she started to scream. Riding on the back of my bike was one thing. Going into a dark, crowded stable with people and horses she didn't recognize was another. Actually, it wasn't another. She didn't go in. She stayed in the entrance and screamed loudly until I decided to put her back in the bike seat and bike someplace else. The screaming, just as I had optimistically calculated, was actually not a problem for these very patient city horses, especially trained and able to keep cool in the company of special-needs kids. But short of dragging Lina into the ring and throwing her up on the horse's back without me being up there already as bait (which they did not allow) there wasn't going to be any horseback riding for Lina. But I wasn't going to give up so easily.

Six months later, I took her to a stable in the north Bronx that had an outdoor ring surrounded by inviting fields and trees. We had been there two years ago, when Lina had been running up and down the fields like she was one of the horses, let out of the barn on the first day of spring. At that time, though, evaluating her suitability for therapeutic horseback riding was out of the question. Stephanie, the very good-natured German evaluator and riding teacher, and I agreed that it would be good to wait a year and reevaluate.

Spring of 2011 seemed like a good time to reevaluate. It was a beautiful Saturday morning in the middle of May. Special-needs students were already riding around the ring, peacefully sitting on their horses, quietly listening to the teacher's instructions. Lina and I walked around saying hi to the horses while waiting for the lesson to be over so that Lina could have her pre-riding assessment, which consisted of walking around the ring, holding the teacher's hand, and accepting a helmet on her head. As we were investigating the area, Lina found a potato chip vending machine. But the machine didn't work. Lina's patience was beginning to run out and when her patience runs out, screaming takes over. And when screaming took over, a young man came out of an office next to the indoor riding ring to tell me to please make the screaming stop. Hoping that people at this stable had gotten the swing of dealing with kids with special needs, I politely explained that making Lina stop screaming was not so easy. The young man explained that unless we didn't immediately leave the premises, the horses would "flip out." The young man was very close to flipping out, but the horses didn't even flip their ears. For me, though, this was all the pre-riding assessment I needed. And honestly, it wasn't as if I expected Lina to score an A-plus in holding the teacher's hand while peacefully and quietly walking around the ring with a helmet on her head. But clearly, riding at this stable was for very special special-needs kids. The ones who would sit quietly and nicely on a horse and didn't get visibly and explicitly frustrated when the vending machine wasn't cooperating.

We walked back over the fields down to the road and hopped on our scooter, long enough to fit both of us, that would take us to the bus that would take us to the subway that would take us home. It was downhill. I had recently figured out that doubling up on a scooter was a dignified alternative to having Lina in the child seat on the back of my bike, which she had outgrown. Riding in front of me on the scooter is also riding, I told myself and kissed my little recently disqualified daughter's soft cheek. I felt thankful that she didn't understand how many programs and treatments and parties and vacations, schools, playdates, concerts, and family gatherings her difficulty to self-regulate has excluded her from.

Sound Therapy

Around the same time, in early May of 2011, we decided to try sound therapy. A year and a half earlier, Lina had been evaluated at the Spectrum Center to see if she would benefit from the Tomatis Method, which uses sound to stimulate the brain. Dr. Alfred A. Tomatis was a French physician and otolaryngology specialist who developed a method of auditory stimulation that enhances the development of language and communication as well as improving learning and behavioral problems. The idea behind sound therapy, according to Dr. Tomatis, is that the ear builds, organizes, nourishes, and balances the nervous system. But with Lina screaming and kicking, refusing to stay in the evaluator's room, even the evaluation that would help determine if sound therapy was for her had been difficult to carry through. So we waited. But when I talked to Dorinne Davis at the Davis Center in New Jersey, she assured me that sound therapy was possible whether Lina would cooperate or not. She would certainly have this optimistic hypothesis tested. It wasn't that Lina was any less active and self-directed in the spring of 2011 than the two previous years. It was just time. And Davis seemed so confident that no matter how much Lina kicked and screamed, their equipment would enable them to evaluate Lina's auditory processing and establish whether Lina would be a good candidate for sound therapies.

Lina did kick and scream. And by the time we left the evaluation, the soil from two giant pots with impressive plants in them was spread all over the fancy rug in the evaluation room as well as on the floor of the elegant lobby. Davis's kind and patient assistant was breaking a profound sweat and Tony was furious at me for having brought Elsa to the appointment and for not having arranged for extra help to deal with Lina while we were trying to understand the complicated auditory theories and how they applied to Lina. Nevertheless, Davis managed to catch glimpses of Lina's red face as Tony and I tried to hold her in the right position and the assistant struggled to keep the headphones on Lina's head. The tone of Lina's own voice, screaming or not, as well as the way her brain processed the sound sequences that were introduced in the headphones was all recorded and, remarkably, we left with our mission completed. Davis had even volunteered that out of the hundreds of kids she had worked with, there had indeed been one boy just as challenging as Lina who was still successfully evaluated and treated. I know this was meant as reassurance but it left me with a curious feeling of having one very special child.

From the evaluation we learned that Lina had certain hypersensitive thresholds, unobtainable acoustic reflexes in her right ear, and that she "processes sound better through bone conduction than air conduction in the vestibular, language, and attention/focus areas." We learned that this processing, through bone conduction, was excessive, meaning that in some ways Lina was too receptive to certain sound frequencies. We also learned from the recording of Lina's voice that "her voiceprint demonstrated many irregular patterns indicative of body imbalances." Based on her findings, Davis recommended three therapeutic sound interventions. Auditory Integration Therapy, Listening Training Programs (such as Tomatis Method), and BioAcoustics therapy to "support her overall wellness with rebalancing irregular patterns of general function such as nutrients, biochemicals, muscular weaknesses, and issues associated with methylation imbalances." I called and scheduled the Auditory Integration Training for the time in August when Lina and Elsa were out of school.

With the summer approaching I fantasized about taking the girls to the summer house in the south of Sweden, which one of my brothers and I had inherited after my mother's death. I knew it was wishful thinking. The sound therapy might have been in the same category—pure fantasy—but if there was a chance that it would contribute to what eventually would make taking vacation trips alone with the girls something more than a dream, then I was all for trying. When summer rolled around, we actually decided to wait further for the Auditory Integration Therapy, until Lina was a little more willing to keep headphones on. Tony started to offer Lina headphones with her favorite music at his place. Lina's teachers asked for headphones for Lina to have on as a reward after completed work. Gradually, Lina became comfortable with the headphones and by November 2011, we were ready. By February 2012, we had figured out the logistics with the Davis Center and Beth, the person at Davis Center assigned to help families who wish to conduct sound therapy from home, traveled to us to teach Tony, Sean, and I how to get started.

We all had our private prejudices for how Lina would react. A few years earlier, I had met another mother, who had told me about sound therapy that she carried through with her son, and I had intuitively felt that this could be an important support for Lina as well. But neither I nor anyone else who knew Lina could have predicted how dramatically and immediately she would respond to these therapeutic musical frequencies as we put the headphones on for the first time. She started cooing. Smiling. Listening intently. Staring into our eyes. Her posture perked up. Her body relaxed. She seemed like someone had just shot a vial of heroin into her vein. We were stunned. The cooing and deep relaxation in response to the weird-sounding songs kept on for the remainder of the two-week program. For the next year, sound therapy became an integral part of Lina's life. I firmly believe that sound therapy has helped Lina to process language more effectively and become more expressive. It is very possible that it also has helped her to transition better from one place or person or activity to the next, and that it, as Dr. Tomatis believed, supported Lina's nervous system in becoming more organized and balanced, helping her to interact more effectively and deliberately with her environment.

ABA with a Relational Approach, an Integrated Model— Round Two: Giving it Another Chance with BOOST

While I was reluctant to go too deep into behavior therapy for Lina at home, both Tony and I agreed to introduce more behavioral strategies by trying out the Jewish Community Center's after-school program for kids with special needs called BOOST. Jennifer Clark, who was one of the leaders at BOOST, recommended children be

accompanied by someone other than their parents when introduced to the program. Sean went with Lina. The first time did not
go so well. Lina screamed at the top of her lungs and wanted to
go swimming at the Olympic-size pool that she considered to be
the most intriguing part of the JCC. But Jennifer Clark, flexible
and brave as her reputation promised, was not discouraged. While
Lina had to leave for that day, Jennifer welcomed her back for
the following meeting, and encouraged us to wean Lina into the
program by first coming by for short periods without the pressure
of registering and see how it went. The next meeting, Lina met
with the group in Central Park, and that evening Jennifer sent a
picture to my cell phone of Lina sitting on a park bench, interacting with another girl! In his notes that evening, Sean described
how Lina had played ball with this same girl, throwing and
catching the ball back and forth ten times! From then on, Lina
was at BOOST, cutting and pasting, practicing circle time and
turn-taking, listening to iPods and playing Zingo, twice a week.
The fact that Lina asked to go there even on days where there was
no after-school program proved her readiness.

Coach Marvin

During the winter break of 2011, I also brought Lina to Coach
Marvin, a gymnastics trainer at a small, Upper West Side gym
working with kids of all ages and abilities, typical and not so
typical. Hanging out in the playground of Elsa's school after
pickup, a mother of one of Elsa's friends, who also has a child
with special needs, was glowing as she described how this coach,
originally a gymnast, had made her daughter enthusiastic about
climbing and jumping, doing pushups and sit-ups, handstands
and somersaults. I called Coach Marvin and somehow knew,

instantly, from the warmth and friendliness of his voice, that we had stumbled upon something good. Thank goodness for mothers. How beautiful it is when mothers get together with their kids running in all directions and yet manage to have meaningful conversations about the essential details of each other's lives. Lina walked into the lobby of the gym for her first day with Coach Marvin, looked closely at the giant, beautiful, black man smiling warmly at her, took his hand, and walked with him into the gym to start her first lesson. He made her climb ropes and ladders, they jumped together on a huge trampoline, she rolled around in tunnels, and she swung around on the barrel like she was born in a gym. And as soon as we left, she turned to me and said, "Can I please have a Coach Marvin!" From then on, whenever summer, fall, winter, and holiday breaks rolled around, Lina would be swinging and climbing and jumping with her beloved coach.

The Public School Option

There are no perfect solutions. No absolutes. No good and bad, right or wrong. Trying to provide Lina with what she needs to help her find the words, connections, imagination, and physical and sensory comfort when she is lost, is the very flexible foundation we stand on. As much flexibility as we have needed in continuously evaluating Lina's after-school work, we needed to keep thinking about her basic education.

Rebecca School was great and we knew how lucky we had been to have had Lina there for two years. But we felt Lina was ready to move on. And when we were presented with the sudden transition from the familiar class and the teacher to a new class at Rebecca School and an unknown teacher, Tony and

I found our opening. The board of education had sent us a letter presenting their yearly offer of a school placement for Lina. This year, it was the Mickey Mantle School on the Upper West Side, a block away from Tony's new apartment and eight blocks away from mine. The first thing Tony and I were struck by as we came to visit was that the kids looked happy. The lower floors had classrooms for kids with learning disabilities and kids on the spectrum. The classrooms on the higher floors were for children with social and emotional issues. Teachers and speech people, occupational therapists, and paraprofessionals, working one on one with the kids who needed ongoing assistance, looked happy, too. Some told stories about having left the school but then missing it so much that they came back. Most of them had been there for long periods and had no intention of leaving. They seemed committed and enthusiastic, flexible and open. There was even a swing hanging from the ceiling in the sensory gym. Tony and I left smiling. After a few more visits, we decided to take the leap. Lina was going to start her summer school in a class of six kids. Ms. Anna Rivera would be her teacher. On the first day of school, with Tony on one side and me on the other, Lina walked up the stairs of the Mickey Mantle School, facing her new adventure with unusual poise. As we were walking through the crowded entrance, a tall lady with short brown hair walked in. I took one look at her friendly, gentle face and asked hopefully, "Are you Ms. Rivera, by any chance?"

"Yes!" she responded and smiled with the kind of warmth and natural openness that made our day—Tony's, mine, and, most importantly, Lina's. As the four of us walked into the crowded but peaceful cafeteria, chatting comfortably, Lina simply sat down with the other kids, opened her lunchbox, and started eating.

Of course, nothing in life is just black and white, and there were many days when Lina hid her head in my arm walking up the stairs to the school in the morning while mumbling her "Mama right here" reassurance phrase that comes up every time I'm about to leave her when she doesn't want me to. If she only knew how I miss her when I am not with her. If only she could see how I risk my life leaning out from my sixth-floor window when she leaves on Fridays to go to Papa's house, just to get a glimpse of her, wandering down the street in her orange shoes, down to the river, next to Sean, to pick some crab apples and do a little swinging in the playground. If she could only watch me after she fell asleep and see how I just lie there, listening to her breathe, wondering what she is dreaming, and looking forward to waking her up and hearing her sweet, "Can I please have a smouch?" A "smouch" is deep pressure against her back, using my body, pressing against hers while she is all wrapped up in a big, thick blanket. A smouch is what we all ultimately want out of life more than anything else, isn't it? Someone who loves us so much that they, with their very real, tangible bodies, hugs us so tightly and firmly and convincingly that all the uncertainty, all the loneliness, all the doubt and the fear and grief just dissipates from our bodies, our hearts, our souls. Lina is just more in touch with this need. She doesn't know how to use language to obscure what is in her heart. In some ways, I feel that this is a much more honest approach to life. Lina is happy if she has the people she loves around her, the food she likes, the swinging in the hammock to great music with the people she cares about singing with her and making sure that the swing keeps on swinging. And now and then going outside to touch the soil, the puddles, the tiny little "apples" on the trees next to the river. And, occasionally, breaking a rule or two in order to connect better with the animated, reddening, shriveled-up faces in the loved ones around who are so curiously invested in not being disobeyed.

So, when we're walking up the stairs to the school, and Lina grasps my arm tightly, repeating her "Mama is right here" mantra, I have to respect where she is coming from. I have to respect it and understand it while simultaneously thinking that life just had mercy on us to introduce us to such a wonderful public school with everyone from the friendly policemen and women in the doorway, making sure that none of the self-directed kids escape out on the street, to the sweet, white, hippie-style speech therapist (not Lina's) who distributes kisses and hugs to all the mothers waiting to pick up their kids, to the older bus driver who calls me sister, to the very approachable assistant principal. With his instinctual understanding of human behavior in general, and special-needs kids specifically, the assistant principal spent no more than five minutes with me and Tony describing Lina before knowing that Ms. Anna Rivera would be the perfect teacher for our daughter.

Early on, Ms. Anna and I had a little one-to-one conference. It was like hanging out with a sister. A co-mother who had all the same concerns and ideas and visions about Lina as the ones that keep me awake at night. I knew, the day when Anna, at drop-off, told me that Lina had made her way into her thoughts during her weekends, that she was a gift to us. I knew, too, by the way Lina took fast little steps over to Ms. Rivera at drop-off, as if her teacher was the person on the other side of a stormy river, welcoming her to overcome her fears, and freeing her to leave me behind for another day at school. Our first parent-teacher conference was like a demonstration in telepathy. We were like two twins sharing the same thoughts about how to relate to Lina's disregulated states at this particular time in her life. Listening to Anna was like hearing myself talk about the desirable balance between understanding and respecting Lina's sensory and emotional needs and making the demands that are just within Lina's reach and would move her to the next level. We laughed at the end of the meeting, Anna and I, about just that, telepathy. This woman was the mother away from home. No wonder Tony had fantasies about marrying her! I shared his enthusiasm. If Tony found someone like her, there would be one more person, a very warm and capable person to love Lina and Elsa.

At the two-thirty pickup, as Lina warmed up to the people around her, they also got to experience many different sides of Lina. In Lina's communication book, I was given reports of Lina's more challenging "moments," as her teacher so respectfully called them, including throwing food on the cafeteria floor, throwing herself on the floor and screaming, or throwing a chair in the classroom when frustrated and overstimulated. There were moments of lateness to the bathroom or lateness in pulling down the pants in time and reminder notes to bring in extra clothing and to remember to wash up and bring back the underwear she borrowed from another girl in the class. There were also notes and stories about Lina's infamous escapades. As usual, Lina would test out her new territories by figuring out how and if she could escape. A little bit like her own personal fire-escape trial, though luckily, Lina was more interested in seeing if she could get to the big auditorium or ride up and down the elevator or make it to a higher floor for a visit with the older kids, than seeing if she could leave the building.

And luckily, if her priorities were to shift during these practice runs, it would be very difficult, even for a Houdini-style little girl like Lina, to escape the police staff that faithfully stood by the door at all hours for as long as the school was open.

The Hammock

The overall picture, whether due to a new phase of development, the spirit world responding to my prayers, the antiviral medication prescribed by Dr. Darrell Lynch, the sound therapy, the BOOST after-school program, or the slightly shifted approach at school or at home, Lina was much calmer. Part of it, I do believe, was that Lina, and everyone around her, over time, developed a better understanding of her very urgent sensory needs.

The day when I put up a hammock in Lina's bedroom deserves to be remembered as the day that significantly improved all of our lives for the next couple of years. The hammock helped illustrate how acutely dependent Lina is on regulating her sensory system on an ongoing basis. What kid would swing in a hammock for hours if their disregulated sensory system didn't beg them to do so? To be with Lina in the playroom, making sure her swing was constantly moving, created opportunities for interaction that had seemed completely unrealistic before. Lina and I had conversations. I asked her to do a puzzle and reassured her that as soon as the puzzle was done, she would be able to go back to the swing and listen to another song. I requested that she throw a ball back and forth with me, and count every throw whether I caught it or she caught it while at the same time maintaining eye contact with me. And for the first time since she was three and a half before losing everything, she did. With the safety of knowing that she soon would be back in the swing where her body and nervous system would feel normal again, she was increasingly able to not just count and throw the ball, but to take pleasure in it! I was thrilled. We listened to music together; we both relaxed. Pushing the hammock was much easier on my back and legs than bouncing on the ball, with Lina wrapped around me. We sang along with the music and just enjoyed each other's company.

In general, Lina would be most comfortable when I sat down next to the swing and pushed her each time she swung my way and sang along loudly with the songs. She liked to hear my voice along with the music. If I stopped, she would soon start whining. It felt like we were back in time, to when she was a baby, lying in the sling that was wrapped around my neck and that both Tony and I used to carry her around in until she fell asleep. From her first month of life up through at least two and a half years old, she would lie in that mini swing, staring into my eyes, listening to me singing, either by myself or along with some CD I put on. And the feeling now, with Lina in the hammock, was so similar. She looked so content and peaceful with only her face visible in the swing as she gazed into my eyes, listening attentively to me singing along to Stevie Wonder, Tracy Chapman, or Sarah McLachlan. It was like magic. It was as if we had suddenly gotten the opportunity to regain some lost ground. One such swinging and singing moment, I got a little carried away, experimenting with harmonizing with one of Lee Ann Womack's songs about love and betrayal. It hadn't been my best performance. Lina, from inside the swing with not even her face peeking out, soberly reviewed:

"Whining!"

With the comfort of the pending return to the womblike existence of the hammock, Lina and I were able to get through whole books together, without tantrums and pages being ripped. We were able to draw and write, sing a full song together by the keyboard, me playing and Lina singing, with the support of the safe containment of the hammock right next to her. I suddenly felt the liberty to push Lina with questions about her full name, her age, address, what she may be feeling and about people in her life without inducing full-blown tantrums. As soon as Lina rose to the challenge, she was immediately rewarded with swing time. I didn't see this as imposing on Lina's own motivation and polluting her integrity with expectations of external rewards every time she did something. I saw it as life and the way we all relate to it. If we didn't know we had a chance to eat or rest or play at some point later, it would be very hard for any one of us to get motivated to work hard. For Lina, who has such trouble holding onto and remembering things in the future, she needed more immediate reassurance in order to feel safe and okay exposing herself to requirements and expectations on the outside.

It was in that same spirit that Lina got things done at her new school. In an email update to me, Tony, and the occupational and speech therapist, Ms. Anna described how she was working with Lina in the classroom during the fall of 2011.

> *It's a little more challenging to provide Lina with the sensory input that she needs in the classroom, but we do try to provide as much as we can by giving tight squeezes, providing a weighted pillow, having her jump. . . . I have learned that when she becomes agitated, one way that seems to work to calm her somewhat is to gain her attention and*

ask her what she wants. Many times, she can tell me. Today it was her apple. So in order to help her participate in group during circle time, I placed her apple near me, but in her view. I asked her to sit quietly in her chair (while she waited her turn with the particular activity) and when she seemed agitated, I reminded her that she was "working" for her apple. Every few minutes, I would let her take a quick bite. . . . She seems to understand the idea of the delay, which makes me feel that this may work for her. I'd like her to feel like she can express her needs and have them met, while still getting her to participate during group instruction and learning new skills that are unfamiliar in the beginning.

Lina began to do really well at her new school. She started to march right into the cafeteria in the morning with a big grin on her face. She would walk right up to the table where her class-mates and teachers sat, put her bag down, take her jacket off, and head straight for the morning cereal line. Saying goodbye to me became an increasingly smooth transition. How different it felt to walk away from Lina's school day in the morning without feeling torn apart by the echoes in my head of her despairing cries for me. Maybe the location of Lina's school added to her ease. It was right in our neighborhood. Maybe she intuited that I would be right around the corner if she needed me. Or maybe she simply liked her new school better than her old one. Maybe the increasingly explicit expectations on Lina, both at home and school, helped make things more comprehensible and calm for her. As usual, these are the things that will keep us guessing until maybe one day Lina can tell her own story. One reason for Lina's seemingly calmer demeanor might also have been that everyone in her environment seemed to be on the same page.

Everyone—Lina's teachers at school, teachers and assistants in her after-school program BOOST, Coach Marvin, Tony, me, and our babysitters—had very specific and explicit expectations of Lina. And while Lina did not always agree with whatever we all wanted her to work on—puzzles, drawing and tracing various shapes, naming colors and things, matching, counting, sitting by the table, singing a song with us from start to finish, following an obstacle course—I think it provided her with a certain sense of safety and a structure that she was ready for at this point.

Without that structure, if it was up to Lina, we would be roaming the parks picking little red and yellow crab apples with her from dusk to dawn.

"Can I please have a apple-picking!" she would ask everyone, everywhere, every moment of the day. It was, of course, a seasonal obsession. Winter and spring didn't produce any apples, but during late summer and throughout fall and into early winter, for as long as there were any apples left on the trees and ground, Lina wanted to be there to pick and smoosh them between her fingers. The softer and more rotten the little apples were, the better the sensation for Lina. If uninterrupted, Lina would stay for hours, focusing only on the trees, scanning every branch for the good, rotten ones that allowed her the full joy of demolishment and annihilation. If no one helped Lina turn the page, she would complete her joy by sliding every other apple into her mouth. She would position herself away from whoever was with her, and slip one in. Talking to Lina about the way these apples are kept colorful and beautiful with pesticides that most likely wouldn't make her feel any better than she already did, was not effective. The only effective measure was to walk away, with Lina kicking and screaming, scratching and punching like the intense fighter she became when she slipped into her autism element. After a few miserable transitions like that, she got the idea. Apples could be smashed in her hands, smeared into her clothing, trampled on, thrown around, and picked endlessly, but they could not be chewed.

To make apple picking a little more productive, I introduced "challenges" for Lina in between the smearing. I had her throw pinecones and pieces of branches at various targets. Every time she hit the target, she was free to go back to her beloved apples. I had her jump and count, run and circle various trees, balance on a big, thick piece of branch that had been blown down after a recent storm. I chased her and tried to entice her to chase me. I made quizzes and asked her to join me in looking and pointing at helicopters circling above us. And she went along with it because she knew if she did she would soon return to her trees. It was the same principle as using the hammock for sensory support that would allow Lina to venture safely into the world of the unknown for a while, reassured that she would soon return to her own preference. Swinging in the hammock one day, Lina sang a joyful song to herself:

"Apple picking, apple picking, makes me smile."

Why does she love it so much? I have asked her a million times but she never answers; she just turns her focus back to the little red apples, scanning the tree for the rotten ones, the ones she can squeeze into her hands or drop on the ground and flatten with her feet. When I was little, there was a kind of hedge by the side of the road on my way home from school that had little inedible berries that made a funny popping sound when you threw them on the ground and smashed them with your feet. I do remember the pleasure of this. Lina's crab apples don't make any sound. They just make a mess in her hand and on her clothes. She looks so free and at peace when she stands there under the little trees by the Hudson River, scanning the branches for more soft ones. She looks like a little farmer, who without any question or reluctance, willingly and in her usual matter of fact way, puts in her hours out on the fields to assure herself that bread is on the table each day. Lina's apples don't put food on the table. They just make her smile.

Sign Language

A friend of mine once asked me why I always stare at people's hands when they talk. It's a good question. Hands express so much. Love, anger, peace, affection. Hands help us accentuate and illuminate language. Hand helps us focus and pay attention. I noticed this in Lina, in particular, because the difference between when she is mentally present or distracted is so dramatic. Whenever I found a way to illustrate with my hands what I was saying, she had less difficulty getting the message. She frequently used the sign for "more," spontaneously bringing her fingertips together in front of her stomach, while at the same time verbalizing what she wanted. "Can I please have some 'chios' [pistachios]," or "Can I please have a swing," were often accompanied with this sign. Whenever I illustrated my words with some kind of gesture, she was more interested in what I was saying. When I moved my hands in front of my face as I spoke to her, it seemed easier for her to engage with me. And she quickly picked up on my gestures, readily adopting them for her own purposes.

I was delighted to make this very simple discovery and went to a bookstore and picked up the most official-looking flash cards of the American Sign Language that I could find. Then I selected a handful of flash cards, illustrating words that Lina currently struggled with or had shown confusion about, such as "not yet," "soon," "tomorrow," and "later." Signs for "happy," "sad," "angry," and "frustrated" would help introduce Lina to and engage her in more abstract communications about feelings and states that so often were expressed only by kicking and screaming. Lina would swing in the hammock in the playroom while I sat on the mat next to her, pushing the swing while trying to come up with relevant contexts for the words we were working on. Whenever the context seemed too contrived and my imagination dried up, there was always the sign for "I love you," fitting into every context. Soon, I added "always" to the "I love you," and while I think Lina has never had any doubt about the validity of this statement, signing while saying it seemed to add to both her comprehension and concentration, somehow making her more available to the meaning of those words.

Our playroom times together were invigorated by this new agenda. "Stop," with the side of my right hand slamming onto the palm of my left hand, had more power than the word alone. "Playing" seemed more fun with my thumbs and little fingers on both hands raised and rotating out and back. When I moved my clawed hands in toward my body with all ten fingers crooked as I illustrated "want" she knew that I hadn't missed the fact that she wanted her vitamins for the third time that day. And even though she couldn't have them, my gestures underlined and clarified that she had been understood. And when my reassurance that she would get her vitamins in the morning was accompanied by resting my left hand inside my right elbow and then raising my right arm from the elbow, showing the sign for "morning," it was easier for Lina to hang onto and take comfort in the idea that she would eventually have what she wanted.

Sign language was an exciting venue because here was something that would help not just Lina but also me and other people in her life to work on words in a more deliberate way, make language more lively and engaging. The signs helped bring us back to that early developmental phase of shared attention so exciting in typically developed kids around the age of one and two. When she had been that age, Lina had been right there pointing and sharing every little detail of her world with a growing number of words. Sign language was now like a new door opening into a room where we had been together before. I think Lina sensed this somehow. Even when we were doing other things, she would pick up the deck of cards that we were currently working on and look at them, going over them, carefully turning the cards over, seeming to know on some level that here was something potentially useful. I got another box of cards for Tony's house, and started to spread the news. Sean started to use them, too. Lina's teacher at school as well as her teachers and assistants at BOOST got lists of words that Lina was currently working on.

Elsa one day asked me, "Mama, why are you always obsessing over the cards these days?" Faithful to my psychoanalytic training, I answered her question with a question. "You think I'm obsessing over it?" She did think so and she was right. While Lina often strikes me as the most present and genuine person I have ever met, she spends so much time in her own world, away from us, shut out from so much shared understanding and shared experiences. My mother once explained to a close friend of mine that she would crawl from mid-Sweden to south of Sweden on her bare knees if that would help my oldest brother with his life, which was very troubled. It's the sort of self-dramatizing thing my mother would say. But I understand the sentiment. And sure, if somehow crawling on my knees from one town to the next would help my children rather than just put me in a wheelchair, I would go down on my hands and knees and start moving. Learning signs is easier. And probably more effective.

The Relationship Between Autism and Reflux

Why is it that good things so often seem to happen almost by accident? Tony and I were sitting in his office one Tuesday morning after having dropped off the girls at school, gearing up for filling out all the initial intake forms describing Lina and the type of treatments and therapies we have tried so far and sending them off to the well-known gastroenterologist Dr. Arthur Krigsman, who specializes in the gut issues of children with autism. We were staring at the pile of forms that looked thicker than *War and Peace*, trying to figure out how to best approach this intimidating process. Tony called Dr. Krigsman's secretary for good ideas about where to start and we were advised to find a good, local MD willing to help us administer all the blood, urine, and stool tests that needed to be completed before we even could talk to the doctor. While Lina's DAN (Defeat Autism Now) doctor, Dr. Lynch, who was practicing up in Northampton, Massachusetts, had helped us administer a lot of tests over the past three years, the extent of this intake process required a local helping hand. Dr. Christina Hift had a reputation of being helpful to many NYC kids with autism. We called and set up an appointment with her, hoping she would be okay with ordering all the tests we needed to consult with Dr. Krigsman.

Tony and Lina and I went to Dr. Hift's office a cold, sunny Saturday morning, a couple of hours before Elsa and I were to sing in a choir for the Swedish Lucia celebration at a beautiful Central Park West cathedral. Lina spent just about one calm minute at the office before all hell broke loose. She didn't want to be there and neither parent's efforts to amuse, entertain, and soothe her made even the slightest dent in Lina's deafening shrieking and throwing whatever she could grab hold of. My attempts to calm her down brought me within the reach of her furious punches and bites. Backing off to give her space resulted in more kicks and screams. She was acting like a rabid tiger and with Dr. Hift coming out into the waiting room and Tony and I interfering in each other's efforts to get the situation under control, things got worse. So I asked Dr. Hift and Tony to go and start the intake interview while I simply sat down on top of Lina's back while holding her hands and flailing arms down like a sheriff calming down a thrashing criminal. Only Lina was not a criminal. She was just stuck and panicky in a world where people communicated with a language she couldn't understand and didn't know how to use. Lina quickly calmed down. It became my turn to try to bring Dr. Hift up to date with how it all happened, what we did about it, and how Lina had responded to our various attempts to help her.

Maybe it was the tension from Lina's outburst, or maybe it was having to go over all the painful details about losing Lina again and again. I don't know what it was, but Dr. Hift annoyed me. However, as she and I were getting increasingly entangled in disagreements about auditory versus visual processing difficulties, I began to notice that actually, this woman seemed to have read a whole lot about treatments and medications that have been tried with kids with autism. She told me she thought it unethical to perform the invasive gastrointestinal radiology recommended by Dr. Krigsman in kids who are already massively invaded before carefully evaluating whether such testing is advised or needed. She told me that she had gone to the Defeat Autism Now (DAN) conferences and has a son, now an adult, who had severe gastrointestinal problems but was now doing well. She also said that she thought Lina's difficulties, from what she had seen and heard so far, were more likely to be caused by upper gastrointestinal issues such as reflux, rather than lower intestinal difficulties. My subsequent pictures of Lina's stool confirmed Dr. Hift's hypothesis that Lina was probably suffering from reflux.

Dr. Hift did not seem the slightest bit impressed by Lina's behavior in the waiting room and told me she had seen much worse. She also commented that she doubted that Lina had autism at all and that the carnosine Lina had been taking to calm down her brain waves and to increase the threshold for seizures may have caused the aggressive behavior. Recent research had shown that many kids on carnosine do well for the first four to five months before the positive effects commonly turn into aggressive behavior. She also informed me that the amount of Valtrex, the antiviral medication Lina was taking, was not a high enough dose to be likely to affect any viral issues Lina may have, while at the same time, she described some potential positive secondary effects of this medication. But Valtrex is a strong medication and not very gentle on an already compromised gut flora. I left the office one hour late to the last rehearsal before the Lucia concerts that were to happen that evening, with a prescription for a serious reflux medication and a sense of excitement about the prospect of working with someone who seemed to be doing her homework. I took Lina off both carnosine and Valtrex, and added the reflux medication Lansoprazole. Lina seemed to benefit. She had fewer outbursts halfway into meals and also seemed to be more comfortable in general.

Simultaneously with biomedical and medical approaches to Lina's well-being, playroom work continued. The more focused, whole-hearted, and enthusiastic time Lina and I, and Sean and Lina, spent in the playroom, the more accessible Lina became to us. While Dr. Hift did not seem very impressed with any of the doctors who had been involved with Lina's care, I almost detected the trace of a smile on her stern face when I described the playroom work to her. Spending a lot of time joining Lina on her terms, and starting every new task with her being solidly engaged, was, and is, the guiding principle.

Homeopathy and Toxicology

And then there was Mary Coyle. A mother of a son with autism who is now flourishing in college, Mary uses the lessons gained from her son's recovery to help other struggling parents. She has dramatically changed the lives of children with autism for over fifteen years. Tony, Lina, and I visited her Manhattan office one warm summer morning in June of 2012. Her office was as bright and cheerful as Mary herself, with her dimples showing and her friendly green eyes and relaxed manners putting everyone at ease. We sat down on the bright yellow couch and learned about how acupuncture, naturopathy, and homeopathy could help Lina's body detoxify and heal itself.

The theory of homotoxicology, developed by the German physician Dr. Hans Heinrich Reckeweg in the 1930s, contains six stages of health. The first three stages are what he termed the "Humoral Phases." This is when the body possesses the ability to "react," through inflammation and excretion, in order to remove invading pathogens and toxins. This includes loose stools, sweat, a runny nose, etc. In essence, the body is able to "fight back" through these reactive responses. The other three phases, termed the "Cellular Phases," are when the body has reached a stage of exhaustion and is having trouble or is no longer capable of "reacting" to the toxic assault. This eventually enables the toxins to penetrate the body on an intracellular level. Once in this deeper phase, according to Dr. Reckeweg, more insidious damage to health occurs. Mary explained how toxins, when they infiltrate a person on a cellular level, lead to a state of degeneration which results in various serious diagnoses such as cancer, diabetes and autism. Helping the body eliminate toxins through the primary pathways, such as the skin, liver, kidneys, and colon—so that the body doesn't have to rely on the secondary eliminative pathways, such as the nose, lungs, stomach, genitals, and bladder—are the goals when working within this model of healing.

In other words, we would now start the journey of helping Lina get closer to a place where she would be able to eliminate the toxins in her own body, in her organs as well as on a cellular level. I looked around Mary's office. There were bottles with homeopathic drops and remedies everywhere. Lina walked around as if she lived there, unscrewing bottles and touching everything on Mary's desk. Mary seemed completely unbothered.

"I want her to like coming here. Let her be, I don't mind," she said, waving away any doubts Tony or I may have had about how much damage Lina might be able to inflict before our consultation was over.

As Mary talked, I looked at Tony, at Lina, and at Mary and thought to myself, "This is an historic day." We had now found what we'd spent years looking for. I didn't understand half of what Mary explained that day. But I was certain this was a woman who could help us with the part of healing Lina that Tony and I couldn't do on our own.

We started on gentle, natural, low-potency herbal remedies to help specific organs to safely remove toxic build-up. Sure enough, we have seen more frequent bowel movement and urinating. There seems to be a positive connection—as Lina continues to remove more toxins through her excretory pathways, her entire system follows suit and relaxes. She walks around smiling and saying "hi" to strangers and friends, holds attention and eye contact much longer, expresses herself much more spontaneously, attempts to take part in conversations around her, and her tantrums are less severe and of shorter duration than they have been for a very long time.

Mary also suggested acupuncture using a low-level cold laser pen. The goal is to balance Lina's acupuncture meridians. The idea is that while helping Lina to calm down from tantrums and outbursts, we would simultaneously induce her with energy through the acupunctural light therapy. Three times a day we would point the light for ten seconds each at various pressure points on her hands, feet, and sides that corresponded to different organs in her body. By increasing her own energy level in this way, Lina wouldn't be forced to apply a tantrum to feel okay. We have seen a big difference.

Mary explained how tantrums, screaming and kicking, and biting and running were Lina's own way to kick life into the shut-down state in her body overwhelmed by toxins, raise her blood sugar to an acceptable level, and stabilize herself.

On Mary's recommendation we have also started to work with Dr. Lawrence Caprio, specializing in allergy detection and treatment. With Dr. Caprio's help we now have a list several pages long of foods that Lina is allergic to, including everything red (from her beloved red apples to red peppers), chicken, and garlic. With "neutralization drops," meant to desensitize Lina to most of what she is allergic to, three times a day, she is doing even better.

Our work with Mary Coyle is still in progress. But already, Tony and I haven't seen Lina doing so well and being so happy, accessible, and harmonious since before her regression into autism. The difference is noticeable to everyone around her. And we have only started our journey of detoxification and desensitization.

HANDLE® Approach

At one of our visits with Mary Coyle, we were discussing neuro-developmental training for Lina. How else can we help Lina to recover what she lost during these difficult years? Apart from regular playroom work, homotoxicology, and allergy treatment, I wondered what the next step was to help Lina slow down and relax enough to process and learn more effectively. She was still more likely to run rather than walk when moving from one room to the next. And while sleeping much better at night and being happier and falling apart much less frequently and severely, she still seemed so preoccupied with making herself feel okay on a very primary level, with very little energy left for focusing on things beyond satisfying basic sensory needs.

"Call Katie Penque," Mary said and handed me her card. "HANDLE Care, Empower to Free," read the card. HANDLE stands for Holistic Approach to Neuro Development and Learning Efficiency. Katie Penque had been working as a volunteer for a Son-Rise family who also used the HANDLE approach to help their son. Seeing how effectively it helped this boy, Katie put her plans to become a psychologist aside and began her training at the HANDLE Institute, founded by Judith Bluestone (author of *The Fabric of Autism*), to become a HANDLE practitioner. In 2009, Katie opened her own practice in the New York Metro area, assisting mostly, though not exclusively, kids with neurological challenges on and off the autism spectrum.

A month later, a very sunny Presidents Day in February 2013, Lina, Valerie, and I stepped into Katie's office to spend the day with her. During the first part of the day, Katie was learning about Lina's challenges and functioning through questions and observations. During the afternoon, Katie presented Lina's neurodevelopmental profile. The basis for her observations was a chart of sensory-motor interdependency and interaction that at first glance looked like a map, tracing the way pigeons prance around in circles, chasing each other, never seeming to rest, never walking in a linear fashion.

All sensory processing systems are intricately dependent on each other, Katie explained. She demonstrated how Lina's constant movements and fidgeting, and her love for the hammock, swinging, and jumping, were her way to compensate for imbalances and processing difficulties in her vestibular system, and that staying still, for Lina, meant feeling queasy and out of sorts. I learned that apart from touch, taste, and smell, which develop during the first two months of an infant's life, all other processing, that is, all other sensory-motor functions, are dependent on healthy vestibular functioning, which becomes fully developed in utero. Being that the vestibular system registers all movement in the body, it serves as the foundation for all other processing, including proprioception (awareness of one's body in space), kinesthetic functions (movement patterns), muscle tone (how one is able to hold up against natural gravity), oral motor function, auditory and visual functioning, receptive and expressive language, and so on.

I learned that Lina's difficulty falling asleep was related to her proprioceptors not sending her sufficient information about where her body is in space, so with the lights out and no ability to jump around to compensate for this lack, she felt completely lost. No wonder she is more concerned with pressure, wanting the pillow and the blanket pressed heavily on top of her, rather than whether she is able to get some air from under all of it! I learned that muscle tone has nothing to do with strength or athletic ability and Lina's low muscle tone puts her in a position where everything she does upright is a constant battle against gravity. No wonder she is always so happy lounging around on the couch and in the swing, in a horizontal position, getting a break from all that force, pulling her down, down.

I learned about Lina's vision: that her eyes do not cooperate and integrate visual information well, making converging difficult, and so Lina is inclined to watch things peripherally, rather than straight on. To look straight on, Katie explained, judging from how Lina uses her vision, is very likely to be an extremely uncomfortable, dizzying, and nauseating experience. All of this and many other challenges make it very difficult for Lina to focus on the faces of others long enough to pick up on their signals.

I left Katie's office with renewed awe of my daughter's ability to smile and be playful, sweet, and affectionate in spite of her massive challenges in every sensory-motor area. Being forced into a kind of fight or flight mode of operating, trying her best to handle all of her overwhelming sensory needs, left very little space for things like focusing on more abstract matters, detoxifying herself, digesting, and picking up on cues in others. As a consequence, expressive and receptive language, attention, and differentiation (using one part of her body without having to employ her whole body), not to mention math, reading, and writing, were falling by the wayside. Equipped with eleven different neurodevelopmental exercises that included tapping, massaging, and tracing Lina's different body parts, as well as an exercise where Lina sucks on a crazy straw and blows little colorful cotton balls around, we drove home with a strengthened sense of mission and a heroine in the backseat.

In all efforts to help Lina have the best life she can possibly have, I believe that the underlying premise is the most decisive factor. Is the foundation of our relationship mutual, or is it not? Do I always remember that Lina, even if she cannot ask for it, is in just as much need of respect and autonomy as someone who could ask for it more explicitly? Am I as interested in and validating her experience whether I understand it or not? When I am present, and when I don't try to protect myself by acting as if I know it all and can control my little girl, emotion and intonation imbues her words. During one of Lina's and my special

Tuesday nights, when it's just her and me, we were lying on the futon, waiting for her to fall asleep. I was thinking about all the sorrow we had been through. All the outbursts and how limited I felt sometimes in knowing how to help my daughter. I talked to her in my thoughts, telling her that I know I'm not perfect, I don't always know what to do, but I'm here, and I love you. "I know," she said out loud and fell asleep.

Afterword: Winter 2016

It's been about three years since I wrote the hardcover edition of this book. Between then and now, I've been everywhere with Lina. In my mind's eye, in my prayers and dreams, I've been to soft sandy beaches and high mountains, I've been in deep forests and open meadows. I've seen Lina skipping happily along naturally bouncy, quiet forest paths, I've seen her dancing with elves and flying with eagles, I've watched her swimming next to dolphins up on the very top of huge waves in green-blue waters. The rational part of me tells me that most of what I've actually done for the past three years is watching Lina walking and skipping along asphalt pavements in New York City parks, flying in the air on upper west side swings and swimming in indoor pools with only the little waves of other swimmers' splashing. We have been New Yorkers for all this time. It's been good, obvious even. But I feel a change coming. Real soil, real waters, trees and mountains.

Lina is twelve now. She is on the cusp of early womanhood. She is hitting it much sooner than I did. I catch myself wishing that it was the other way around. She seems so unprepared for her body to change. With yet so few words to describe something as big as adolescence, a rapidly changing body, a fluctuating mind, a whole new intriguing territory. And yet, Lina, more than anyone else, has helped me understand that wishing for other things is like getting the best present this life can offer and throwing it away without opening it; without fully figuring out what the gift was.

Lina showed me that whatever I can think up, whatever I imagine that I want out of my life, is nothing compared to what I can have if I receive everything as it is. I look at my twelve-year-old pre-adolescent and think that she must be the most beautiful person God let on this earth. With that vastness in her eyes; that quiet, deep, non-manipulative, ego-less, unassuming, and perfectly authentic presence, she brings me back to the incredible mystery and awesomeness of every minute on this planet.

I have come to believe that challenge can bring a huge opportunity. No, I am not going to try to convince anyone or myself that it feels wonderful to have one's illusion blown into a thousand pieces. I am on this earth, like most humans, with all my tendencies, all my reactions, obsessions, possessiveness, insecurities. But Lina's autism taught me that if I can somehow learn that losing and winning, darkness and light, are variations of the same basic thing, then I can stop with my endless, anxious categorizing of all things in life as either good or bad, desirable or undesirable, welcomed or unwelcomed, and start living fully in what *is*. Most of us have our whole lives wrapped around a number of illusions that we justify until we're blue in the face— whether that is: the one person we can't see ourselves losing; the child that can't be anything other than what we expect him or her to be; our life's work not going as we expected it to go. . . . Then we have our most cherished illusion blown out from under us into little, untraceable particles that we can never piece together again no matter how much we try. As we're sitting there, in the rubble of our broken dreams, we have the unique opportunity to wake up a little. To see that actually, our unhappiness has nothing to do with us not getting what we want. It's our *clinging* to our illusions that makes us unhappy, unhealthy, insecure, unfocused, and non-present. The bust is the first step towards our own real life. What happened to Lina was a big bust for me, as well as for her father and sister.

Lina's language disappearing, her incontinence, the raging unsettlement in her body, the difficulties to create and maintain friendships with other children. . . all of it, was shocking, disintegrating, mind-blowing. Finding a way to relate to it all was almost as difficult as finding Lina. Both are ongoing processes. Lina is doing so much better. She is calmer, more comfortable in her own body, her language continues to evolve and is slowly, very slowly, becoming more and more an expression of her rather than an echolalic imitation of others.

Thanks to Lina, I have become an Anat Baniel Method® NeuroMovement® practitioner, trained by Anat Baniel who studied and collaborated with one of the first neuroplasticians, Moshe Feldenkrais. For the last year and a half, I completed the basic training and am now in the middle of the children's mastery training, all the while giving Lina NeuroMovement lessons every chance she gives me. The central idea of NeuroMovement® is that our brain is an Information System that seeks to put order within all of our environments. Movement is the main source of information to the brain that helps the brain to grow, form, and organize itself. In turn the brain then gains the ability to organize all of our movements, thoughts, feelings, and actions and to lead us from the seemingly impossible to the possible, to healing.

Lina knew from the start that there was something to this method. Tony had contact with Anat Baniel via his publishing company. I had read Anat's book *Kids Beyond Limits* where she describes her work with children with special needs and the 9 Essentials that makes her work so unique. Anat was in town for a conference a few years back. It was a beautiful spring day when Tony and Lina and I walked into her hotel room on 59th street, Central Park South, for a meeting that eventually changed all of us. She was an attractive lady, much smaller than I had imagined her, with reddish-brown curls. She looked at me, at Lina, at Tony, with strong, piercing and yet loving eyes, and somehow I instantly knew we had found someone who could help us. Tony and I tried to describe what brought us there while keeping track of Lina who was soon full-on jumping on Anat's hotel bed and kept asking for the elevator, while munching on, and spilling, banana chips all around the room. Eventually, Lina moved a little closer to Anat, standing next to her and staring, unabashed, right at her. Anat just kept on talking with Tony and me, seeming completely unaffected by Lina's close up investigation. Lina has always had a special place in her heart for people with a strong personality. Anat, with her un-modified Israeli accent, and a kind of certainty in every word she let out that bore witness of an unusual intellectual clarity, a willingness to take responsibility for what she knows and express it without a trace of ambivalence, was no doubt someone who also possessed a strong personality. Soon, Lina stood even closer to Anat, now checking out her wild curls, her long straight nose while looking right into her eyes.

At some point Anat turned to Lina and started talking to her, discussing Lina's favorite subject, food, and whether she was hoping to get more banana chips or bean chips later, or maybe something more interesting, like cake? Anat began to touch her very gently on her shoulders, her ribs, her legs and feet, her pelvis and sternum all the while she kept conversing with her about all the food that makes this world good. It was such a subtle touch and yet so acutely present that Lina forgot about going to the elevator. She forgot about us. She forgot about all the restlessness that had rushed through her blood just a few minutes ago. She was completely still. Didn't say a word. Didn't move at all. I watched her turn all of her attention, not to Anat but to herself. I was witnessing magic. Warm tears flowed down my cheeks as I watched my daughter find herself. Anat looked over at me and smiled. "You're crying." "Yes of course." I said, "I have never seen anything like this." After the lesson, Anat and Lina walked out on 59th street, hand in hand, as if they had known each other for a whole lifetime.

The summer came and we went to Anat's center in San Rafael, California, to have her and her associates work with Lina for two intense weeks. During that time, Anat said to me, "I don't really want to do this to you but I'm afraid I'm going to do it anyway." "Do what?" "I know your life is full the way it is. And you don't need more. But I think you should take the training." I looked at her no less bewildered as I was amused. Was she kidding? How would that work? Would I bring the girls? Would I leave them?! The training involved weeks and weeks away from Lina and Elsa, something I had quite simply never done before. Part of it was online and long-distance, but most of it was in-person, intensive, ten day–long segments, spread out over the course of fourteen months. It seemed like an almost ridiculous idea and I basically just felt like I humored Anat by saying I would think about it.

It became much more than a ridiculous idea. And as I have completed the basic training, I'm now in the middle of the next phase, The Children's Mastery. I am hooked. Or maybe more correctly, I am unhooked. I feel free. Open. Like anything is possible. And I am curious about the magic of NeuroMovement. Curious about what Lina is going to say or do next.

She is speaking more and more, her own words, putting together her own simple sentences, showing more and more of her own personality. She has developed an interest in people's colors and it's becoming increasingly clear to anyone who knows about auras that Lina actually can identify them on most people that she meets. She catches jokes. She even makes jokes: Pretends that Nicole, the clinical director at ATLAS is Brian. As Nicole tries to clarify, Lina laughs, happy about her own ability to have intentional impact in social situations. And Lina herself doesn't get flustered as easily as before. She can handle that it will be a few hours before she gets to go in the blue car with me or a couple of days before a celebration with the cinnamon buns she loves or a few more months before it's warm enough for her to swim in the ocean. I can take Lina with me now to Fairway, the supermarket around the corner from our house, without turning the whole place upside down. Last week on Valentine's Day, Lina showed her deliberate intention to connect with her little sister by wanting to send pictures of herself to her. We are continuing with homeo-toxicology with the guidance of incredible homeo-path and director of the Real Child Center, Mary Coyle; we also carry on with biomedical interventions as suggested and overseen by integrative pediatric neurologist Dr. Maya Shetreat-Klein. We are doing more sound therapy as well as collaborating with Amanda Friedman and Alison Berkley, the loving and inspired directors of Lina's new downtown school Atlas. And now, for this past year, we have added NeuroMovement to Lina's life.

Life is calmer and less complicated. We all have time to take deep breaths and think about what we want to do next in our lives together as well as in our individual lives. I have time to think about writing my next book. And this book will not be about autism, though in some ways, everything I do from now on has something to do with autism, something to do with what Lina taught me during those very challenging, constantly illuminating years.

Lina falls asleep by herself now. After the swinging in the hammock and listening to music, singing along together, talking about her day, people and their colors, reading "What is Love" or "How do Dinasours Say I'm Mad" or "If You Give A Pig A Pancake" a couple of times each. There is the time when she wraps her blanket over her head and turns her tall, slender preadolescent body away from me, with the "leave the door open" comment that unmistakably means that she wants me to go about the rest of my day someplace else. So at this cue, I turn out Lina's little wooden lamp next to her bed, kiss her forehead and cheek, tell her how happy I am to have her here with me and how very much I love her. Then I say goodnight, and do as instructed. I leave the door open and lay down on my own futon in my own room next to hers. Occasionally, she would let out a "yeah" in acknowledgement. Up until recently, autism has held back anything beyond that, in those emotionally charged situations. It would be easier for Lina to comment on things that were a little further away from her, in time and space. She would say "I want to see my Papa" to everyone else but Tony and "I want to see my Mom" to everyone else but me.

So for years, "good night" and "I love you was on me." I wouldn't dream of asking her to say any of it back. I would not ask of her that she assimilate anyone else rather than expressing something from her own heart. The very thing I want to help Lina find for herself is her own spontaneous and authentic expression, not just another form of social echolalia and more scripted sentences that she already has so much of.

So I continued my little night time procedure with what was. But then one night Lina said "goodnight Mom" back. It was almost shocking. I did not know what to do, so I stood there in the doorway, staring at her. Gradually, her saying "goodnight Mom" became no big deal. It was really nice to hear but it no longer left me speechless. Then one night, after I spilled my heart to her like a hundred thousand times before, she said, "I love you Mom." There is nothing like those three words for a mother or a father or a sister or a brother from a kid who has trouble talking. If a thousand knights on white horses were riding up to me and telling me from the bottom of their hearts that they indeed loved me for all the right reasons, that still would be nothing but a pee in the Nile compared to Lina's quiet "I love you Mom." It was an experience of everything being alright. Of course I know that everything would be alright even without these words. I'm just so human. I went into my room and just sat there on my futon, blinking, wondering if I was dreaming. From her room, as if she wanted to make sure I really got it and wasn't going to start doubting it, messing with it in my own insecure mind, she said it again, and again, and again, about 20 more times. Maybe she too had been waiting to find those words. Maybe she had also felt some kind of joy in formulating what is, no doubt, the most important words existing in the human vocabulary. I don't know. All I know is that life with Lina will never stop being interesting. I don't know what is to come or where she will go or who she will be, but I know that whoever has been close to her during these very colorful years, has learned not just to survive, but actually enjoy, some pretty wild weathers.

Buddhist monk Pema Chodron, in Wisdom of No Escape, describes how *renunciation* has to do with being open to the present moment instead of being trapped by a kind of misguided nostalgia for wanting to stay protected in what we know, even if it's limited and petty. For me, one of the invaluable lessons from Lina's autism was and is about learning how to open and soften rather than shutting down and harden in the face of challenge. Pema Chodron describes how the ravens in Cape Breton near her monastery loves the wild weather.

> *The wilder the weather is, the more the ravens love it. They have the time of their lives in the winter, when the wind gets much stronger and there's lots of ice and snow. They challenge the wind. They get up on the tops of the trees and they hold on with their claws and then they grab on with their beaks as well. At some point they just go into the wind and let it blow them away. . . they are hardy and fearless and playful and joyful; the elements have strengthened them. [p. 54]*

More than anyone I have ever met, Lina helped me see that whatever I think I want out of life; if I can let go of that; lose it; laugh at it; play with it; be light-hearted about it, while still working for and keep moving towards what I believe in, then I can be free and fearless like the ravens. Then I too can get a glimpse of the vastness, the pure, raw, unlimited energy that fills up every single moment of this beautiful life.

About the Author

Helena Hjalmarsson, M.A., L.C.S.W., L.P., is a psychoanalyst in private practice in New York City. Her practice is informed by the idea that everything is interconnected, the healing powers of true acceptance and belief in living in the now. She is the co-author of *The Quotable Book Lover* and is published in *Psychoanalytic Social Work* on "Transference Opportunities During the Therapist's Pregnancy: Three Case Vignettes." She has published multiple articles in Swedish newspapers and magazines. Helena is also an Anat Baniel Method®–NeuroMovement® Practitioner, trained by Anat Baniel, who studied and collaborated with Moshe Feldenkrais. Helena lives in New York City with her two daughters, Lina and Elsa.